Manual Therapy for the Prostate

Manual Therapy for the Prostate

Jean-Pierre Barral,
DO, MRO(F), RPT

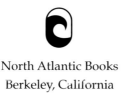

North Atlantic Books
Berkeley, California

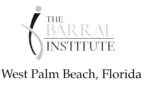

West Palm Beach, Florida

Published by   and
North Atlantic Books   The Barral Institute
P.O. Box 12327   8380 Woodsmuir Drive
Berkeley, California 94712   West Palm Beach, Florida 33412

Cover image © iStockphoto.com/skahlina
Cover and book design by Brad Greene
Printed in the United States of America

Manual Therapy for the Prostate is sponsored by the Society for the Study of Native Arts and Sciences, a nonprofit educational corporation whose goals are to develop an educational and cross-cultural perspective linking various scientific, social, and artistic fields; to nurture a holistic view of arts, sciences, humanities, and healing; and to publish and distribute literature on the relationship of mind, body, and nature.

North Atlantic Books' publications are available through most bookstores. For further information, visit our Web site at www.northatlanticbooks.com or call 800-733-3000.

Library of Congress Cataloging-in-Publication Data

Barral, Jean-Pierre
    [Manipulations de la prostate. English]
    Manual therapy for the prostate / Jean-Pierre Barral.
        p. ; cm.
    Originally published as: Manipulations de la prostate / Jean-Pierre Barral. c2005.
    Includes bibliographical references and index.
    Summary: "Written for manual therapy practitioners, this book presents an alternative to more drastic prostate medical treatments"—Provided by publisher.
    ISBN 978-1-55643-900-1
    1. Prostate—Diseases—Treatment. 2. Manipulation (Therapeutics) 3. Osteopathic medicine. I. Title.
    [DNLM: 1. Prostatic Diseases—therapy. 2. Manipulation, Osteopathic—methods. WJ 752 B268m 2010a]
    RZ371.B37 2010
    616.6'506—dc22
                                                          2009045987

1 2 3 4 5 6 7 8 9 UNITED 14 13 12 11 10

Contents

Introduction

For the osteopath or manual therapist, the human body is an indivisible and indissociable whole whose components are indispensable to homeostasis and good health. Each articulation, every organ and tissue deserves our care and attention.

Sooner or later, nearly all men have prostate problems. The urinary, genital, and psychoemotional consequences are not conducive to a good quality of life. Thanks to these simple, effective, and noniatrogenic techniques, precise manual therapy can help to resolve the effects of prostate problems.

This book is the fruit of everyday clinical experience. Based on anatomy and physiology, *Manual Therapy for the Prostate* provides a simple response to a complex pathology. As you will see, the techniques are not aimed at reducing the size of an adenoma but rather to improve the extensibility, Mobility, Motility, and compressibility of the prostate.

It is a practitioner's duty to help the many patients who have benign prostatic hypertrophy. This book is one of the keys to bringing them some relief.

Chapter 1

Anatomical Review

The Prostate

The word prostate comes from the Greek word prostates, from proïstanai, meaning "placed in front" or "to be exposed." This is most likely because the prostate is located in front of the rectum. It will be shown that on the emotional level "to be exposed" has a particular significance.

The prostate weighs just under an ounce, but its "social weight" becomes increasingly heavy. It is estimated that 30 percent of men will undergo prostate surgery before age eighty.

In some cases, osteopathy or manual therapy can be of great help to patients suffering from prostatic adenoma. Surgery and medications carry with them many iatrogenic effects, including impotence and incontinence. It is our duty, to whatever degree possible, to assist these patients in avoiding surgical intervention.

Appearance
Shape

The prostate has the form of a chestnut, like a flattened cone. Some describe it as having the heart shape seen on playing cards.

Consistency

The prostate is firm, smooth, and elastic to the touch, a bit like the distal part of the thenar eminence or a somewhat ripe pear.

Size

The size of the prostate varies a lot with age. In young men, it measures:

- 1.2 inches (3 cm) vertically
- 1.6 inches (4 cm) across
- 1 inch (2.5 cm) in thickness

External Configuration

The prostate is flattened from front to back (fig. 1.1).

- Its base is cranial.
- Its apex is caudal.
- Its ventral surface is flat and vertical.
- Its dorsal surface is transversely flat and vertically convex.

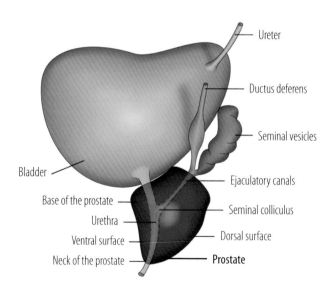

Figure 1.1. External configuration of the prostate.

It displays a shallow median sulcus and two lateral lobes. It is this posterior surface that has the shape of a playing-card heart. It is important to be able to palpate the middle groove, as its disappearance indicates that the prostate has increased in size.

Internal Configuration

The urethra and the spermatic pathway traverse the prostate. The prostate is described in relationship to these structures:

- A ventral prostate, or isthmus, lies in front of the urethra.
- A cranial prostate is situated behind the urethra and above the ejaculatory ducts. This part is *estrogen dependent;* it is where adenomas develop.
- A caudal prostate is located posterior to the urethra and inferior to the ejaculatory ducts. This part is *androgen dependent;* it is where prostate cancer is found.

Structure

Stroma

The prostatic stroma is made up of connective tissue and smooth muscle fibers. The prostate is enveloped in a fibrous capsule that firmly adheres to it. Around the capsule is the periprostatic sheath (de Retzius) made up of concentric tissue layers derived from the pelvic fascia and imbedded with venous canals. It can be envisioned like the outer shell of a chestnut.

The Glandular System

Glandular substance makes up 66 percent of the volume of the prostate, while muscular tissue represents just 33 percent. Within it are about forty tubulosaccular glands that form canals connected together by areolar tissue and supported by fibromuscular trabeculae. These excretory ducts open onto approximately fifteen prostatic sinuses on the floor of the urethra.

The glandular system is divided into periurethral and prostatic glands proper.

Periurethral Glands

As their name indicates, these periurethral glands surround the urethra and are separated from the internal prostatic glands by the external urethral sphincter. These glands are mainly situated on the lateral and dorsal aspect of the prostate. They are particularly concentrated:

- at the level of the seminal colliculus.
- at the level of the bladder neck.

Prostate Glands

The prostate glands are arranged around the lateral and dorsal surface of the urethra. They lie outside the smooth sphincter of the urethra. The urethra is the structure that receives prostatic secretions.

Lobes

The dorsal prostate comprises a left and a right lobe, both of which are stimulated by the male hormones. Between these two areas is the middle lobe, which responds to female hormones.

The ventral part of the prostate contains fewer glandular structures than are found in the rest of the organ. In the luminal surfaces of the glands are small calculi about 0.04 inches (1 mm) in diameter.

Topography
Location

The prostate is very deeply situated in the lesser pelvis between the base of the bladder and the deep transverse perineal muscle (fig. 1.2). It lies:

- beneath the bladder.
- about 0.8–1.2 inches (2–3 cm) behind the pubic symphysis.
- in front of the rectum.

Surrounding it are the genitovesical vascular pedicles.

The prostate surrounds the urethra and the two ejaculatory ducts. For this reason any increase in volume or hardening of the prostate causes a narrowing or a compression of the urethra.

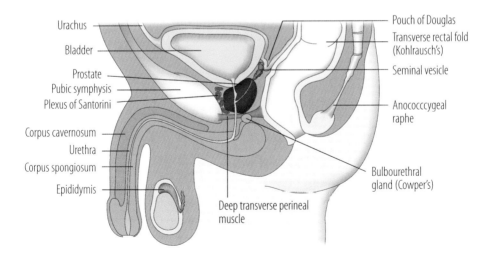

Urachus
Bladder
Prostate
Pubic symphysis
Plexus of Santorini
Corpus cavernosum
Urethra
Corpus spongiosum
Epididymis

Pouch of Douglas
Transverse rectal fold (Kohlrausch's)
Seminal vesicle
Anococccygeal raphe
Bulbourethral gland (Cowper's)

Deep transverse perineal muscle

Figure 1.2. Location of the prostate.

The Prostatic Compartment

The prostatic compartment (fig. 1.3) refers to the pelvic tissues closely surrounding the prostate. It is made up of:

- ventrally, the pubic symphysis.
- dorsally, the prostatoperitoneal aponeurosis.
- laterally, the levator ani muscles.
- caudally, the middle perineal aponeurosis.
- cranially, in front by the pubovesical ligaments and caudally by the trigone and neck of the bladder.

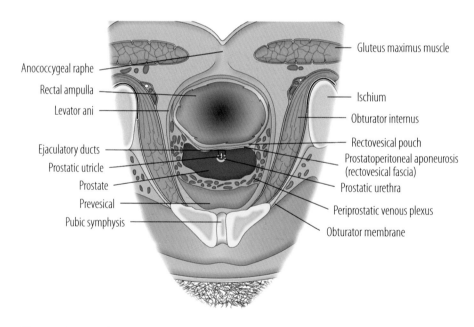

Figure 1.3. Prostatic compartment.

Periprostatic Aponeuroses

The periprostatic aponeuroses surround the seminal vesicles, the vesicle neck, and the prostate. These fasciae are made up of fatty connective tissue containing muscular fibers as well as neurovascular structures. This aponeurosis tissue forms the hypogastric fibrous sheath surrounding the organs of the lesser pelvis. Note that the hypogastric sheath is thicker where it contains neurovascular structures, most certainly to protect them. Around the prostate, from the distal part of the seminal vesicles and the vesicle neck, the hypogastric sheath becomes condensed.

The rectoprostatic (Denonvilliers's) fascia is located behind the seminal vesicles of the prostate. It contains a thin bed of fat and numerous muscular fibers, mainly concentrated at the base and the apex of the prostate. Ventrally and laterally, the hypogastric sheath fuses with the capsule of the prostate. Imbedded in the ventral part of the sheath are the afferent veins from the venous plexus of Santorini. Here it is called the preprostatic aponeurosis of Zuckerland.

From the internal surface of this sheath, the prostatic capsule is continuous with the numerous fibromuscular septa that enmesh the glandular acini.

Implications for Manual Therapy

It is known that fasciae that have muscular fiber components react to mechanical manipulation. They are very responsive to manual Listening Techniques. This phenomenon exists in numerous female pelvic structures, in particular the uterosacral ligaments. *The periprostatic structures have the same property.* It is thought this is because of their regional and central proprioceptive connections.

Caudal Wall of the Compartment

The region between the two ischiopubic rami, the pubic symphysis, and the rectum is called the urogenital diaphragm. Sometimes it is referred to as the perineal floor. It is described in three parts:

- the arcuate pubic ligament
- the transverse perineal ligament (Henle's)
- the middle perineal aponeurosis

Ventral Compartment Wall

This wall is less well delimited than is the dorsal side. There is a slender preprostatic tissue that Farabeuf named the ischio-preurethro-prostatic leaf.

Note that this leaf gives fibers to the neck of the bladder, some of which are continuous with the prevesical umbilical aponeurosis.

Dorsal Compartment Wall

The compartment is enclosed by the rectoprostatic (Denonvilliers's) fascia. This fascia is made up of muscular and connective tissue measuring 0.1 inches (3 mm) in thickness. It is located above the middle perineal aponeurosis. It extends from one levator ani muscle to the other, between the lateral prostatic aponeuroses.

This fascia separates the rectum from the prostate, and it is first in line when manipulating via the rectal route. Note that as it extends upward, it ensheathes the seminal vesicles and the terminal part of the ductus deferens. Cranially, it is connected to the peritoneal floor as it merges with the pouch of Douglas. Some authors think that this musculoaponeurotic lamina is equivalent to the broad ligament in females on account of its rich supply of smooth muscle fibers.

Lateral Surfaces

These are the sacro-recto-genito-pubic aponeuroses that run from the sacrum to the posterior surface of the pubic symphysis. These thick fibrous sheaths are embedded with veins and adhere to the prostate. They contribute in large part to the support of the bladder and the rectum.

Implications for Manual Therapy

The lateral surfaces of the prostate are important to manipulate because of the presence of smooth muscle fibers, and also on account of the hypogastric nerve plexus that give this region heightened sensitivity. It is certainly the nerve plexus that allows the practitioner to obtain a central reaction and a feedback effect on manipulation.

In cases of benign hypertrophy, these lateral surfaces become more rigid. Frequently one side is more affected than the other. Testing their Mobility and extensibility is a key step in the manual therapy evaluation of the prostate.

Cranial "Wall"

The prostate adjoins quite directly with the bladder. Without any partition per se, the bladder rests squarely on the prostate. This contact is a factor in the support of the bladder.

Periprostatic Space

In conclusion: the prostate is not directly in contact with the walls of its compartment. The periprostatic space is laden with cellular tissue rich in smooth muscle fibers. This surrounding tissue forms a sort of fibromuscular vascular shell, which is reinforced laterally and readily palpable by rectal examination.

Prostatic movement in the sagittal plane is more pronounced. Recall that the ventral space is separated from the pubic bone by the venous plexus of Santorini. This plexus of veins allows the prostate to be more mobile anteriorly and facilitates a fairly smooth return movement.

Stability

The prostate is kept in place by:

- the attachments of the prostatic capsule with the fibrous connective tissue sheath external to it.
- its adherence to the base of the bladder.
- its association with the urethra.

Important Relationships

For the principal relationships of the prostate, first the extrinsic relationships and then its intrinsic associations will be studied.

Extrinsic Relationships
Ventral Associations

The prostate is located 0.8–1.2 inches (2–3 cm) behind the inferior border of the pubic symphysis. It is in contact with the fascia of the external urethral sphincter and covered by the periprostatic sheath.

Lateral Associations

The lateral prostatic laminae are fibromuscular extensions of the levator ani muscles that join the prostate. The inferior hypogastric plexus is situated fairly high toward the seminal vesicles.

To reach the inferior hypogastric plexus, direct your fingers as far laterally as possible toward the cranial zone of the prostate.

Dorsal Associations

The prostate is closely related to the rectum, from which it is separated by the prostatoperitoneal aponeurosis. This aponeurosis is also referred to as the rectoprostatic fascia or as Denonvilliers's fascia. Between the aponeurosis and the prostate is a space corresponding to the two leaves separating the aponeurosis. This space allows a surgeon to lift away the posterior surface of the prostate. It is via the anterior surface of the rectum that the dorsal aspect of the prostate is manipulated. Here several things should be readily palpable by digital examination: the two lobes, the median groove, the rounded edges, size, consistency, and Mobility of the prostate.

Caudal Relationships

The neck of the prostate relates to the perineum. It is situated about 1.2 inches (2 cm) behind the pubic symphysis and 0.8–1.6 inches (2–4 cm) below an imaginary horizontal line running through the caudal part of the symphysis. Thus the neck contacts the urogenital diaphragm.

The middle perineal aponeurosis extends between the two ischiopubic rami at their posterior part. It is made up of two fibrous layers surrounding a muscular sheath formed by the two deep perineal muscles. These two muscles are separated by the perineal body. This central tendinous body receives fibers from the anal sphincter, the bulbospongiosus and the two deep perineal muscles, and from the superficial transverse perineal muscle. Depressing the perineal body provides a good idea of the general tone and firmness of the perineum.

Cranial Relationships

The base of the prostate is divided in two slopes by a transversal crest. The dorsal slope relates to the genital structures, while the ventral part is contiguous with the bladder.

Dorsal Part

At its summit, the prostate connects to the seminal vesicles and the terminal ductus deferens. To effectively manipulate the prostate, it becomes clear that it is important to emphasize precise features like the seminal colliculus. This is the elevation in the floor of the prostatic portion of the urethra where the seminal ducts enter.

The seminal vesicles are obliquely placed superior to the prostate and lie flattened against the posterior surface of the bladder. Together with the ductus deferens, they are surrounded by a dense cellular tissue and by the cranial part of the prostatoperitoneal aponeurosis of Denonvilliers. At this level, the aponeurosis of Denonvilliers is very rich in muscular fibers. Early anatomists thought that this fascia constituted an interseminal muscle capable on contraction of evacuating the contents of the seminal vesicles. These fibers certainly play a role in ejaculation and orgasm, which empties them. The pouch of Douglas extends over the seminal vesicles about 0.6 inches (1.5 cm) from the base of the prostate.

Ventral Part

The trigone of the bladder rests on the middle lobe of the prostate.

Intrinsic Relationships
With the Prostatic Urethra

The urethra runs almost vertically through the prostate from its base to its apex, where it becomes more posterior. Its length is about 1.2 inches (3 cm) with a lumen of 0.2 inches (0.5 cm). As it descends through the prostate it forms a gentle curve that is concave anteriorly. At the junction of the tube's superior one-third and the inferior two-thirds, the urethra dilates and becomes the prostatic sinus. In the middle part of the urethral crest is the seminal colliculus, a rounded eminence of 0.4–0.6 inches (1–1.5 cm) in length (fig. 1.4). At the superior part of the urethral crest are two shallow depressions named the prostatic sinuses. They run upward toward the posterior lip of the bladder neck. *For manipulation purposes, this small surface is one of the zones of great importance for the prostate. It will be discussed further in the "Manual Approach" chapter.* The floor of the prostatic sinus is perforated with about fifteen small orifices through which the prostatic secretions flow.

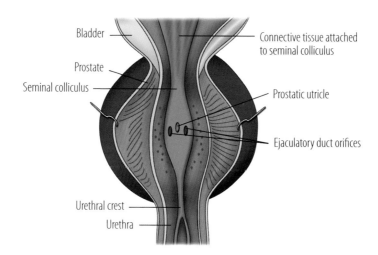

Figure 1.4. Seminal colliculus (verumontanum).

With the Internal Urethral Sphincter (Sphincter Vesicae)

The smooth sphincter surrounds the origin of the prostatic urethra. It is more slender caudally than cranially. Its height is about 0.2 inches (0.6 cm) with a thickness of 0.4 inches (1 cm). It has continuity with the circular musculature of the trigone of the bladder and ends at the level of the seminal colliculus.

With the External Sphincter (Sphincter Urethrae)

The striated sphincter closely surrounds the intermediate part of the urethra, at the neck of the prostate. The neck is the apex of the prostate, where it meets the middle perineal aponeurosis at the urogenital diaphragm. This sphincter constricts the urethra and allows for voluntary control of urinary continence. Its contraction also creates a compression of the prostatic glands at the moment when sperm fills the prostatic sinus.

The prostatic secretion protects the spermatozoa with alkalinity and supplies them with the zinc and fructose essential to their function.

With the Ejaculatory Ducts

The ejaculatory ducts, one on the left and one on the right, stem from the union of the ampulla of the ductus deferens and the duct of the seminal vesicle. The two ducts convey the sperm into the urethra.

Dimensions

- length: 0.7 inches (1.8 cm)
- diameter: 0.6 inches (1.5 cm); the ducts diminish in size toward their terminations, where they measure no more than 0.2 inches (0.5 cm).

Relationships

Above the base of the prostate, the ejaculatory canals run free for several hundredths of an inch (several millimeters) until they enter the prostate. On reaching the seminal colliculus, they diverge around the prostatic utricle. In most cases, the two ejaculatory canals open with a single orifice on either side of the utricle. The ejaculatory ducts and the utricle occupy the center of a common canal that shapes the prostate.

Palpation of the Prostate

The prostate is palpable through the rectal route; this is described in detail in Chapter 4. Its main axis is not vertical but inclines from cranial to caudal and from dorsal to ventral, following an angle of about 20 degrees. It is firm to the touch and not very mobile laterally. Normally the two lateral lobes, and the shallow median sulcus that marks them, should be readily palpable.

Arteries

Branches of the internal iliac artery supply the inferior vesical and middle rectal arteries. They border the prostate cranially and posteriorly.

Veins

Although "the rule of the artery" is one of the fundamental principles of osteopathy, it is the venous system that is of utmost importance here. The prostate bathes in a venous system:

- Anterior to the prostate are the veins of the urethra, the bladder, the plexus of Santorini, and the veins of the bulb of the penis.

- Posterior to the prostate are the hemorrhoid veins. In the chapter devoted to manipulation, a local technique for the hemorrhoid veins is described.
- Surrounding the sides of the prostate are the periprostatic veins.

All of these veins help keep the prostate in place and are shock absorbers for the numerous microtraumas the prostate is subjected to, given its caudal position.

Lymphatics

The prostate vessels terminate chiefly in the internal iliac and external iliac lymph nodes. This network is more developed dorsally.

Sacral Nerves and the Hypogastric Plexus

Presacral Nerve

The origin of this nerve is continuous with branches from the abdominal aortic plexus. These flat and condensed fibers make up the connective tissue cord of the presacral nerve, commonly referred to as the superior hypogastric nerve. The presacral nerve divides into two branches, in the form of an inverted Y on either side of the median line. They descend to surround the rectum as the hypogastric nerves.

Each hypogastric nerve is 3–4 inches (8–10 cm) in length and runs down into the pelvis, gliding under the lateral peritoneum of the rectum. They reunite with the hypogastric plexus between the rectum medially, and the hypogastric vein laterally.

Hypogastric Plexus

The hypogastric plexus (fig. 1.5) is a sagittal cluster of nerves that spreads out in a fanlike fashion. It measures 1.2–1.6 inches (3–4 cm) in the anterior to posterior direction and has a height of 0.8–1.2 inches (2–3 cm). The plexus lies in the extraperitoneal connective tissue and adjoins:

- laterally, the internal iliac vessels and their branches and tributaries.
- medially, the side of the rectum, the ductus deferens, and the ureter.
- caudally, the pelvic floor.
- dorsally, the sacrum.
- cranially, the side of the rectum.
- ventrally, the dorsal wall of the bladder and the seminal vesicles.

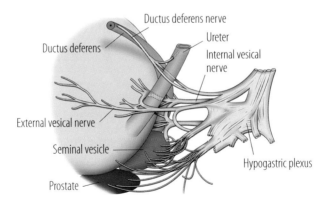

Figure 1.5. Hypogastric plexus (adapted from Testut).

Anastomosis

The hypogastric plexus forms an anastomosis (fig. 1.6):

- with the lumbar sympathetic chain; with the last lumbar ganglion and the sacral chain, notably the second and third ganglions.
- with the sacral plexus; with the third and fourth pairs of sacral nerves that form the pudendal plexus.

Efferent Branches of the Hypogastric Plexus

The efferent branches of the hypogastric plexus innervate:

- the rectum.
- the bladder.
- the prostate (by 5–6 relatively large filaments, distributed posterolaterally).
- the ductus deferens.
- the seminal vesicles.

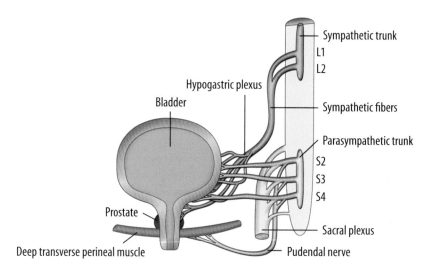

Figure 1.6. Anastomoses of the hypogastric plexus.

In order to optimize the effect of manipulation of the prostate and of the entire urogenital system, the nervous system must not be neglected. The hypogastric nerves are reached via the rectum, placing the index finger onto the cranial and lateral aspects of the prostate. It is rarely felt distinctly under the fingers; the sensitivity of this plexus better confirms correct finger placement.

The Seminal Vesicles

Each of the two seminal vesicles secretes an alkaline fluid that mixes with the sperm as it passes into the ejaculatory ducts. The secretion also contains fructose, vital to the optimal functioning of the spermatozoa. Somewhat pyramidal in form, the base of the seminal vesicles is in a cranial and lateral direction.

Aspects

Dimensions

The seminal vesicles have the following dimensions:

- 2–3 inches (5–8 cm) in length;
- 0.6 inches (1.5 cm) in width.

Consistency

The seminal vesicles are softer than the prostate.

Implications for Manual Therapy

This difference in texture is important here; it tells the practitioner if the manipulations are specifically addressing the prostate or the seminal vesicles. The consistency of the seminal vessels is similar to the feel of a slightly ripe fig. Early anatomists likened their firmness to that of the junction between the bone and the cartilage of the nose.

Topography

Orientation

The seminal vesicles are situated in the frontal plane, lying between the fundus of the bladder and the rectum. They are obliquely placed superior to the prostate. Their main axis assumes a 20- to 30-degree angle directed superiorly, posteriorly, and laterally in relation to the base of the prostate.

Location

The seminal vesicles are enveloped in the prostatoperitoneal aponeurosis of Denonvilliers (fig. 1.7). Remember that this rectoprostatic fascia is very rich in smooth muscle fibers and venules. However, the seminal vesicles themselves are not surrounded by a capsule of smooth muscle fibers.

Implications for Manual Therapy

As previously explained, tissues with smooth muscle fibers react especially favorably to Listening and Induction techniques.

The fibers of the rectoprostatic fascia join the prostatic capsule, whose fibers are continuous with the smooth muscles of the stroma. This is not the case with the seminal vesicles, and therefore manipulation has less proprioceptive effect. On the other hand, it is thought that manipulation of the seminal vesicles may have a *hormone-stimulating action*.

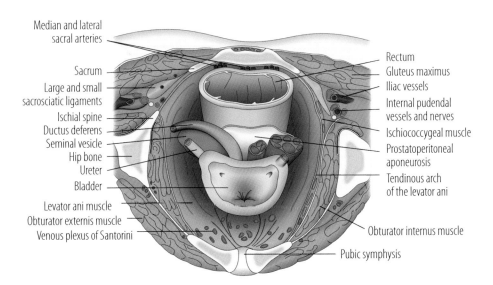

Median and lateral sacral arteries

Sacrum

Large and small sacrosciatic ligaments

Ischial spine

Ductus deferens

Seminal vesicle

Hip bone

Ureter

Bladder

Levator ani muscle

Obturator externis muscle

Venous plexus of Santorini

Rectum

Gluteus maximus

Iliac vessels

Internal pudendal vessels and nerves

Ischiococcygeal muscle

Prostatoperitoneal aponeurosis

Tendinous arch of the levator ani

Obturator internus muscle

Pubic symphysis

Figure 1.7. Location of the seminal vesicles.

Prostatoperitoneal Aponeurosis

The prostatoperitoneal aponeurosis (rectoprostatic fascia) has already been discussed, but it is very important for these techniques that it be examined further. This sheath has a quadrilateral form:

- its *cranial border* fastens onto the vesicorectal pouch of Douglas.
- Its *caudal border* is linked to the middle perineal aponeurosis, after covering the dorsal surface of the prostate.
- Its *lateral borders* joins with the sacro-recto-genito-pubic aponeurosis, more significantly in their caudal aspects.

The seminal vesicles and their fibrovascular surroundings constitute a frontal partition that divides the lesser pelvis into:

- a ventral vesicoprostatic division
- a dorsal rectal division

Connections and Mobility

The seminal vesicles are fixed to the base of the prostate. They can be mobilized in the anterior-posterior and lateral directions. Remember that the prostate is less mobile in the lateral direction. The seminal vesicles follow the movements of the bladder and the rectum.

Important Relationships

- Ventrally: with the posterior surface of the base of the bladder
- Dorsally: with the anterior surface of the sacrum
- Caudally: with the base of the prostate
- Cranially: with the pouch of Douglas; here the peritoneum partly covers them.

Innervation

Innervation is provided by the hypogastric plexus.

Veins

The seminal vesicles are surrounded in a rich venous plexus relating to all the veins of the lesser pelvis.

Implications for Manual Therapy

To manipulate the prostate and the seminal glands, it is necessary to consider the hemorrhoid veins and the liver. There is no satisfactory treatment for hemorrhoids without taking an interest in the liver and diet of the patient.

Palpation

Palpation of the seminal vesicles is performed rectally following the lateral borders of the prostate in a cranial direction. With practice, you will easily be able to feel the difference in firmness between the prostate and the seminal vesicles. Another indication that you are palpating the seminal vesicles is that they have far greater Mobility and compressibility laterally when compared with the prostate. This will be discussed in detail in Chapter 4.

The Rectum

Internal prostate manipulations are all done via the rectal route. It is important to study the rectum and its adjacent structures to become familiar with its characteristics as well as its precise topography.

The rectal compartment is limited in front by the prostatoperitoneal aponeurosis, and cranially, rather loosely, by the peritoneum. The prerectal space separates the dorsal surface of the seminal vesicles and the prostate from the ventral surface of the rectum. Caudally, the space is delimited by the union of the rectum and the pelvic floor, at the caudal part of the prostatoperitoneal aponeurosis.

Important Relationships

The bottom of the pouch of Douglas meets the superior border of the prostatoperitoneal aponeurosis of Denonvilliers. Laterally, the pouch of Douglas is limited by the folds extending from the bladder to the rectum. These folds correspond to the female uterosacral ligament. They are not as strong or elaborated in the male but nevertheless contain some smooth muscle fibers.

Implications for Manual Therapy

As these lateral folds of the pouch of Douglas have smooth muscle fibers, they are important to manipulate. Remember once again that as soon as you are dealing with ligaments composed of smooth fibers, the Listening and Induction techniques work more subtly and more effectively.

Location

In an adult with an empty bladder, the pouch of Douglas is found about 0.4–0.6 inches (1–1.5 cm) from the base of the prostate. It is approximately 2.4 inches (6 cm) above the anus, making it accessible by rectal palpation.

Extraperitoneal Part

The peritoneum is related only to the upper two-thirds of the rectum. Below the pouch of Douglas, the anterior surface of the rectum is linked, on the midline, with the vesical part contained between the two ductus deferens. This is called the interdeferential triangle. The two sides of the triangle are formed by the ductus deferens; the prostate is its summit, and the pouch of Douglas is its base. At the level of the two superior angles of the interdeferential space, the ureters cross the ductus deferens, descending anteriorly and medially.

With an empty bladder, the triangle is 0.8 inches (2 cm) in length; with a full bladder, 1.8 inches. Here the bladder is closely linked to the rectum, from which it is separated by the prostatoperitoneal aponeurosis.

Conclusion

By way of the rectum, you can palpate:

- the prostate;
- the bladder;
- the seminal vesicles;
- the ductus deferens;
- the ureters.

The Inguinal Canal

Testut always contested the name of this canal, which suggests it is merely a pathway to be taken by the spermatic cord and the musculonervous framework that surrounds it. It is a very important canal in so far as it is possible to penetrate it, and with one finger, directly affect genital nerves.

Location

The inguinal canal lies just superior to the medial half of the inguinal (Poupart's) ligament, which is a folded border of the external oblique muscle.

Direction

The inguinal canal follows the oblique direction of the crural arch from cephalad to caudad, from lateral to medial, and slightly dorsal to ventral (fig. 1.8).

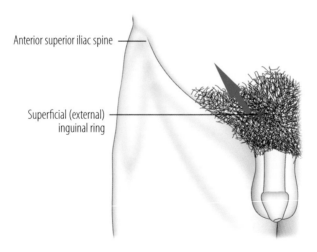

Figure 1.8. Direction of the superficial opening of the inguinal canal.

Dimensions

The inguinal canal is about 1.6–2 inches (4–5 cm) in length. Its width is variable based on an individual's morphotype and tonicity.

Formation of the Inguinal Canal

The inferior insertions of the external oblique, internal oblique, and transversus abdominis muscles will be examined to understand the elaborate nature of the canal.

External Oblique Muscle

The aponeurosis of the insertion of the external oblique terminates at (fig. 1.9):

- the *superior fibers* end at the linea alba.
- the *inferior fibers* arise from the anterior superior iliac spine.

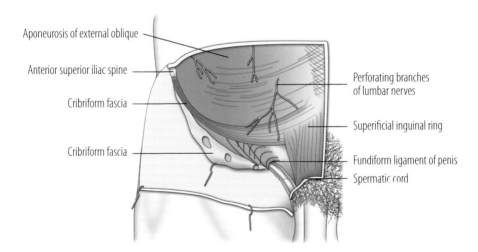

Figure 1.9. Formation of the inguinal canal. Superficial view.

They are directed downward and medially to form a fibrous band called the crural arch. This folded band is reinforced by fibers from the aponeurosis of the iliac fascia. Other fibers form a bridge over the femoral vessels. They are reflected from ventral to dorsal and cephalad to caudad, and they attach to the pecten pubis. This reflected ligament is known as Gimbernat's ligament.

The *middle fibers* are directed toward the pubis. These external superficial fibers run on the spine of the pubis, and some fibers interlace with their corresponding opposite fibers.

The *group of deep fibers* known as Colles's ligament (posterior crus) extend to the opposite side to attach on the pubis and the pectineal line.

The inferior muscular fibers of the internal oblique arise from the ventral lip of the iliac crest and the lateral two-thirds of the crural arch (fig. 1.10). The muscle fibers end in the aponeurosis of the internal oblique, which arches downward and medially, and blends with

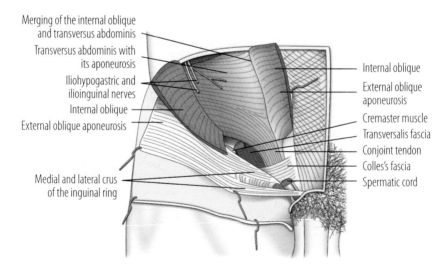

Merging of the internal oblique and transversus abdominis
Transversus abdominis with its aponeurosis
Iliohypogastric and ilioinguinal nerves
Internal oblique
External oblique aponeurosis
Medial and lateral crus of the inguinal ring

Internal oblique
External oblique aponeurosis
Cremaster muscle
Transversalis fascia
Conjoint tendon
Colles's fascia
Spermatic cord

Figure 1.10. Formation of the inguinal canal. Deep view (adapted from Testus).

the aponeurosis of the transversus abdominis muscle to attach to the pecten pubis and the pubic crest. Beneath the inferior border of the internal oblique, the outermost fibers of the cremaster muscle are apparent.

Transversus Abdominis Muscle

The inferior fibers arise from the anterior superior iliac spine and from the lateral thirds of the crural arch. They curve caudally and medially together with the aponeurosis of the internal oblique to attach to the crest and pecten of the pubis, forming the conjoint tendon.

Conjoint Tendon

The conjoint tendon is the common tendon of the lower fibers of the internal oblique and transversus abdominis muscles (fig. 1.11). Its inferior insertion relates to the pubic symphysis, and to the part of the pubis contained between the crest and the pecten of the pubis.

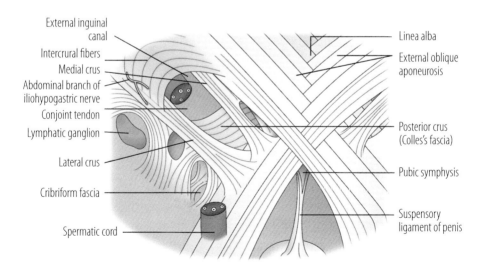

Figure 1.11. Conjoint tendon.

Transversalis Fascia

The transversalis fascia is continuous with the iliac fascia. At the internal inguinal orifice its fibers extend into the canal and descend toward the scrotum to form an envelope for the spermatic cord and testes.

At the crural ring, the transversalis is fixed to the crural arch and adheres to the femoral vessels. It is reinforced by several ligaments:

- the ligament of Henle
- Hesselbach's ligament
- the iliopubic tract (deep crural arch)

Peritoneum

The peritoneum is spread across the dorsal surface of the abdominoinguinal region. At the caudal part of this area, it is reflected to cover the internal iliac fossa slightly above the merging of the transversalis and iliac fasciae. In this area the peritoneum is quite free, except at the superior lateral part at the internal inguinal orifice. This adherence is due to a fibrous cord, the processus vaginalis—a vestige of the peritoneal diverticulum that traversed the inguinal canal during the descent of the testes.

Components of the Inguinal Canal

The inguinal canal has two walls, a roof, and a floor.

Ventral Wall

This wall is thick and strong anterior-posteriorly. It is formed from the aponeurosis of the external oblique, subcutaneous tissue, and by the skin throughout. The anterior surface of the spermatic cord is bordered by the cremaster muscle fibers.

Dorsal Wall

This wall is weaker. It is formed mainly by the transversalis fascia reinforced by the Hesselbach's triangle, the ligament of Henle, Colles's fascia, and the conjoint tendon. The section bordering the internal canal opening is more resilient, and the internal part of the inguinal canal is made sturdier by the conjoint tendon that occupies it. However, between the two is an area of relative weakness. Intestinal pressure is enough to bulge out the dorsal part of the inguinal canal. This is the weak point of the inguinal canal, where hernias occur.

Caudal Border (Floor)

This is formed by the superior surface of the inguinal ligament where it attaches to the pubic crest. This is the medial part of the crural arch.

Cranial Border (Roof)

The cranial border is formed by the arching fibers of the internal oblique and the transversus abdominis muscles.

Orifices

The inguinal canal has two openings.

- A superficial opening called the external inguinal orifice; it relates to the skin.
- The other is called the deep or internal inguinal orifice; it is intimately related to the peritoneum.

  Each opening is surrounded by a ring.

Via the internal opening of the inguinal canal, manual therapy can have a significant effect on the peritoneum. In the case of postsurgical peritoneal adhesions, you can clearly feel a unilateral fibrous tension that is strongest at the internal inguinal ring. It can be either homolateral or contralateral in compensating.

All operations create accompanying adhesions to a greater or lesser degree. On questioning patients, you realize that various types of hernias (inguinal, hiatal, or umbilical) very often appear several months or even years following a surgery. These hernias can be located far from the surgical site. The adhesions and retractions destabilize the reciprocal tension system, and the natural weak points are what give way.

External Inguinal Ring

Location

The external inguinal ring is the exit from the inguinal canal. Oval in shape, its long axis follows an oblique course from cranial to caudal, and from lateral to medial. Also referred to as the superficial inguinal ring, the external inguinal ring (fig. 1.12) is located superior-lateral to the pubic tubercle. It is surrounded:

- laterally, by the lateral crus. The external oblique attaches to the pubis by two tendinous bands of fibers that divide to form the lateral and medial crus. The lateral crus inserts into the pubic tubercle and the body of the pubis.
- medially, by the medial crus, which attaches to the pubic symphysis.
- cranially, by the intercrural arched fibers.

caudally, by the posterior crus or Colles's fascia, formed by the fibers of the external oblique muscle coming from the opposite side.

Dimensions

The superficial inguinal ring measures 1 inch (2.5 cm) in height and 0.4–0.6 inches (1–1.5 cm) in width. *The index or middle finger can enter it easily,* which gives direct access to the nervous system contained in the inguinal canal.

Characteristics

When the abdominal muscles contract, the superficial inguinal ring tightens markedly. Therefore, before a finger is introduced, the patient must have relaxed abdominal muscles, the head placed on a pillow, and one leg flexed. In exploring the inguinal canal, you can ask the patient to contract his abdominal muscles to evaluate their caudal resistance.

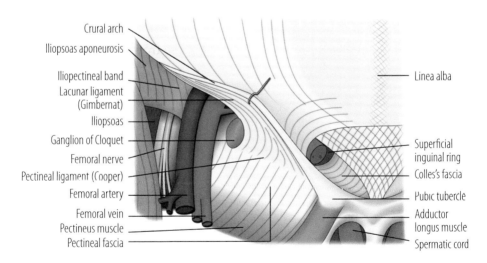

Figure 1.12. Superficial inguinal ring.

Internal Inguinal Ring

Location

The entrance to the inguinal canal is located midway along the crural arch, 0.5 inches (1.25 cm) above and about 2 inches (5 cm) lateral of the pubic tubercle, and 2.8 inches (7 cm) from the linea alba.

Dimensions

The diameter of the internal ring is large, on the order of 0.4–0.6 inches (1–1.5 cm). By engaging a finger in the external inguinal opening and pressing the abdominal tissues in the medial direction of the internal inguinal ring, you can manipulate the peritoneal attachments at their ventral part.

Contents of the Inguinal Canal

The main occupant of the inguinal canal is the spermatic cord, which is composed of:

- the ductus deferens;
- the deferential artery;
- the spermatic artery;
- the testicular and cremasteric arteries;
- an important venous network that on the left flows into the left renal vein and on the right enters the inferior vena cava;
- the lymph vessels of the testes;
- sympathetic nerve filaments.

All of these structures are contained in a fibrous sheath of the transversalis fascia. In the fibrous sheath are the genital branches of these nerves (fig. 1.13):

- iliohypogastric;
- ilioinguinal;
- genitofemoral.

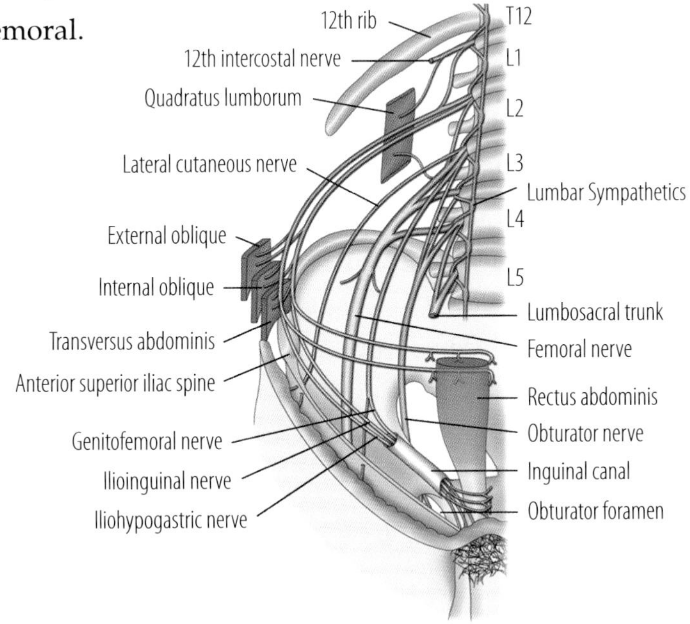

Figure 1.13. Nerves of the inguinal canal (adapted from Testus).

Embryology of the Inguinal Canal

Until the seventh month in utero, the two inguinal rings sit face to face, and the inguinal canal scarcely exists. Later, following the transverse enlargement of the pelvis, the internal and external orifices move apart. The inguinal canal, which was previously oriented nearly anterior-posteriorly, grows in length and becomes oblique.

From the sixth to the ninth month the testicle, which was intra-abdominal, moves into the inguinal canal. It exits by the external inguinal opening and descends into the scrotum. In the course of this migration, it carries with it a peritoneal envelope called the tunica vaginalis.

Up until the ninth month, by which time the testicle has taken up its final position, the two peritoneal tunicae vaginalis communicate via the vaginoperitoneal cavity. When the descent of the testes is complete, this peritoneum lining the inguinal canal fuses, closing off communication with the abdominal layer. However, it leaves its trace as a fibrous cord called the vaginal ligament. At birth, the obliteration of the vaginoperitoneal canal is more or less definitive.

One month after birth more than 75 percent of infants have an obliterated canal. The external inguinal dimple is the only vestige of this canal in the adult. The closing off of the canal may be incomplete; retaining a connection with the general peritoneal cavity is a predisposing factor to some hydroceles and inguinal hernias.

The Female Inguinal Canal

The female inguinal canal contains the round ligament of the uterus, along with the iliohypogastric, ilioinguinal, and genitofemoral nerves. Having smaller contents, the canal is narrower than in the male. However, it is about 0.4 inches (1 cm) longer. The fact that it is not as wide explains in large part why fewer hernias occur in females.

The Cremaster Muscle

This muscle accompanies the length of the spermatic cord.

Location

- Proximally (fig. 1.14): the lateral part of the muscle originates midway along the inguinal ligament as a continuation of the internal oblique muscle. The medial fascicle arises from the pubic tubercle and from the lateral iliac fascicle that inserts onto the femoral arch in the inguinal canal, close to its internal orifice.

■ Distally (fig. 1.15): the cremaster fibers extend as far as the tunica vaginalis, where they more or less envelop the testicles.

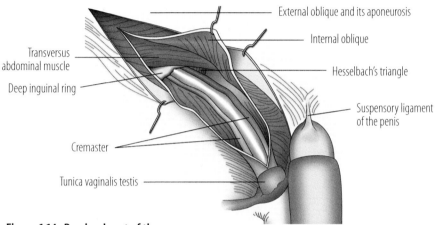

External oblique and its aponeurosis

Internal oblique

Transversus abdominal muscle

Hesselbach's triangle

Deep inguinal ring

Suspensory ligament of the penis

Cremaster

Tunica vaginalis testis

Figure 1.14. Proximal part of the cremaster (adapted from Helga Fritsch and Wolfgang Kuhnel).

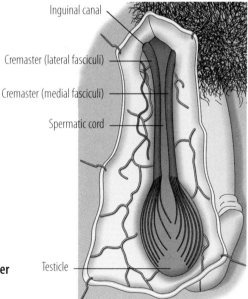

Inguinal canal

Cremaster (lateral fasciculi)

Cremaster (medial fasciculi)

Spermatic cord

Testicle

Figure 1.15. Distal part of the cremaster (adapted from Testut).

Function

The cremaster pulls up the testes toward the superficial inguinal ring. Its contraction raises the internal pressure of the testicles and the epididymis, facilitating the migration of the sperm in the ductus deferens.

The Abdominal Muscles

Transversalis Fascia

The extension of the transversalis fascia becomes the internal spermatic fascia.

External Oblique Muscle

The aponeurosis of the external oblique muscle makes a minor contribution to the formation of the cremaster fascia.

Internal Oblique and Transversus Abdominis Muscles

The cremaster muscle is a continuation of these muscles. Some caudal fibers of the internal oblique leave the inguinal canal and are attached to the spermatic cord to descend with it toward the scrotum.

This chapter emphasizes the interdependence of the muscles of the abdomen, the inguinal canal, and the testicles. Manipulation of the inguinal canal certainly helps to reestablish favorable intraductal pressure in the testicle, the epididymis, and the ductus deferens. It is also believed that this manipulation affects hormonal balance.

The Ductus Deferens

The excretory apparatus of the testicle looks like a long canal. The ductus deferens is a continuation of the duct of the epididymis. Distally the ductus deferens joins with the duct of the seminal vesicles to become the ejaculatory canal (fig. 1.16).

Dimensions

- Its length is 20–24 inches (50–60 cm).
- Its diameter is a minimum of 0.12 inches (0.3 cm).

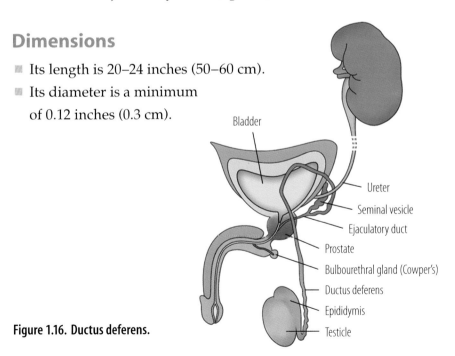

Bladder

Ureter

Seminal vesicle

Ejaculatory duct

Prostate

Bulbourethral gland (Cowper's)

Ductus deferens

Epididymis

Testicle

Figure 1.16. Ductus deferens.

Pelvic Part of the Ductus Deferens

The pelvic part of the ductus deferens runs from the deep inguinal ring of the inguinal canal downward to the base of the prostate. At its start the ductus deferens is cylindrical in form. At its terminal part the canal flattens, widens, and becomes less regular to form the ampulla that receives secretions from the seminal vesicle. Beyond the seminal vesicles, the ductus deferens passes though the prostate as the ejaculatory canal. Along its pelvic course, the ductus deferens measures more than 8 inches (20 cm).

Important Relationships

- In its lateral vesicle part, the ductus deferens lies in the cellular tissue that separates the lateral surfaces of the bladder from the levator ani. It is covered in peritoneum.
- Posterior to the bladder, the ductus deferens is connected to the homolateral seminal vesicle and lies in a double fold of the prostatoperitoneal aponeurosis.

Functions

The vas deferens has a fairly firm consistency, owing to the thickness of its muscle wall relative to the size of its lumen. It has the texture of cartilage. The muscular strata are varying spirals, longitudinal and coiled in form. They play an important role in the intraluminal pressure of the ductus deferens by matching the pressure and thus enabling the spermatozoa to pass through as rapidly as possible.

Both in the masculine and feminine genital systems, pressures in the various conduits are changeable to facilitate the swiftest possible transport of the ovum and sperm. Intraductal pressure gradients vary from moment to moment in response to mechanical, chemical, hormonal, and psychological influences. These stimuli trigger the circular musculature to enact the best response possible in the subtle process of fertility.

Ejaculatory Ducts

Each ejaculatory duct (fig. 1.17) is formed by the union of an ampulla of the vas deferens and a duct of the seminal vesicle. They converge to open on the seminal colliculus via slit-like apertures alongside the prostatic utricle. They measure 0.8–1 inches (2–2.5 cm) in length with a width of 0.06 inches (0.15 cm) at their origin, diminishing to 0.02 inches (0.05 cm) at their termination. Needless to say, the slightest spasm or obstacle can perturb the passage of sperm.

The ejaculatory ducts are situated almost entirely in the substance of the prostate as they run obliquely from cranial to caudal, and from dorsal to ventral. Manipulation of the prostate gland itself has an effect on the ejaculatory ducts.

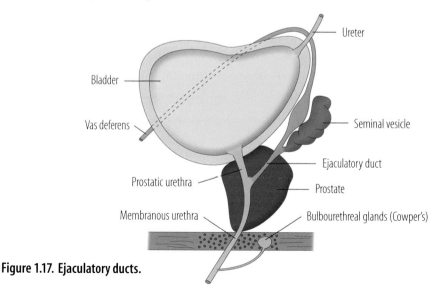

Ureter

Bladder

Vas deferens

Seminal vesicle

Ejaculatory duct

Prostatic urethra

Prostate

Membranous urethra

Bulbourethreal glands (Cowper's)

Figure 1.17. Ejaculatory ducts.

Implications for Manual Therapy

There are no specific techniques for the ductus deferens. An effect can be obtained through the intermediary of the prostate (especially the seminal colliculus) and through the seminal vesicles.

Chapter 2

Functions of the Prostate

The prostate plays a fundamental role in the composition of sperm and in the protection of the spermatozoa when they travel from the vagina to the uterine tube.

These are its principal functions and its contributions to:

- *Visceral mechanics:* the prostate contributes greatly to the stability of the organs of the lesser pelvis, notably the bladder, which rests upon it. It provides this role because of its firmness, its attachments, and its venous system.

- *Urinary continence:* owing to its position and to its relationship with the smooth and striated urethral sphincters, the prostate allows a man to be continent.

- *Excretion:* the prostate produces a cloudy alkaline aqueous solution, containing, among other things, acid phosphatase. This alkaline media contributes to the makeup of seminal fluid in providing it sufficient volume.

- *Secretion:* the prostate secretes an enzyme responsible for the fluidity of sperm. This is called the prostate-specific antigen (PSA). PSA levels are important in cancer detection.

- *Fabrication of fertile sperm:* the prostate is just one of testosterone's targets, along with muscles, hair, libido, and erections.

- *Spermatozoa nutrition:* the prostate extracts zinc from the blood. For optimal functioning, spermatozoa require fructose and zinc. The prostate provides spermatozoa with these two vital elements.

43

It could be said that the prostate contributes to the potency and speed of sperm, as without enough speed they would all be destroyed before reaching the ovum.

■ *Protection from vaginal acidity:* sperm has a pH of about 8.3. It is made up of secretions from the epididymis, the seminal vesicles, and the prostate. One ejaculation represents about 3.5 cc of sperm; 1 cc contains 60–120 million spermatozoa. These motile male gametes are protected from the acidic environment of the vagina (pH = 4) by their own alkalinity (resulting from the prostatic excretion), cervical mucous, and the superior regions of the female reproductive tract.

■ *Opposing retrograde ejaculation:* the seminal colliculus prevents retrograde ejaculation. This rounded eminence on the posterior wall of the prostatic urethra is made up of erectile tissues. When erect, they expand to tip forward. This stops the escape of urine at the time of ejaculation and counters the regurgitation of the semen into the bladder.

Recall that the prostatic utricle, with a length of about 0.5 inches (1.2 cm), is a slit-like aperture situated at the top of the seminal colliculus. It runs superior and posterior in the substance of the prostate between the two lateral lobes and terminates between the ejaculatory ducts, which open onto it. As discussed below, one of the major problems following prostate surgery is the systematic occurrence of retrograde ejaculation.

Chapter 3

Pathology of the Prostate

Statistics on prostate dysfunction vary among authors, but all agree that they represent a genuine threat to men. Presently, averaging the statistics, it can be assumed that 30 percent of men will suffer urination problems before the age of fifty. Beyond age fifty, half of all men will likely experience benign prostatic hypertrophy.

Osteopaths and manual therapists will encounter prostate complaints with increasing frequency. Even as standard treatments advance, they can entail especially serious iatrogenic effects, including impotence and urinary incontinence. Chapter 4 explains that these techniques are not at all harmful. At worst, they simply have no effect on symptomatology.

The various prostate problems are:

- benign prostatic hypertrophy
- cancer
- prostatitis

Benign Prostatic Hypertrophy (BPH)

Definition

Benign enlargement of the prostate is a neoproliferation of stroma and glandular tissue involving new divisions of the glandular ducts. The resulting prostatic adenoma means the prostate becomes enlarged and can, if it projects toward the bladder, compress the prostatic urethra and impede the passage of urine.

Note that it is not the size of the adenoma that defines pathology but rather the functional problems it causes. For example, an adenoma could project mainly toward the rectum without creating any particular disturbance.

In dealing with an enlarged prostate, it is necessary to know how to determine its degree of firmness. Increased hardness is what generates a rise in periprostatic pressure. This pressure will eventually compress the urethra, particularly when the anterior part of the prostate that become fibrotic. *Fifty percent of men with benign prostatic hypertrophy have no symptoms.*

Therapeutic Conclusions

Frequently in this profession, practitioners want to prove their effectiveness with modern investigative means. Ultrasound can reveal prostate size, *but manual manipulation has little effect on volume.* Manual therapy results pertain to the firmness of the prostate as well as to the Mobility of the gland and surrounding tissues. What objective test could evaluate these parameters?

Characteristics of Benign Prostatic Hypertrophy

- Benign prostatic hypertrophy is characterized by the appearance of microscopic nodules in the stroma of the prostate, around the periurethral glands.
- It is the most common benign tumor found in men.
- It does not become cancerous.
- It can present very early, between age thirty-five and forty. Around this age, there is a natural enlarging of the prostate.

Causes

Many theories have been advanced with no formal proof. At present, urologists favor the hypothesis of an underlying *hormonal imbalance* due to advancing age. However, paradoxically, BPH is arising earlier and earlier.

Hormonal Imbalance

The prostate is a hormone-dependent organ governed by androgens and testosterone. When an imbalance occurs between these hormones, the prostate increases in size. Ninety-five percent of androgens in circulation are produced in the testicle under the influence of the pituitary gland, induced by the hypothalamus. Five percent of male hormones are of adrenal origin. Note that the prostate does not secrete any hormones.

Predisposing Factors

Age

As stated above, BPH strikes increasingly early.

Stress

Even if it is not the direct cause, stress can exacerbate symptoms considerably.

Ethnicity

African Americans and Icelanders have the largest percentage of prostatic adenoma.

Genetics

There is increased risk of BPH in a family where a case previously exists.

Sexual Activity

Most authors maintain that there is no relationship between BPH and sexual activity. My experience leads me to question this assertion. After all, men have a tendency to exaggerate their level of sexual activity. It is common in surveys for the lowest response to be that they have had only one sexual connection in the past three months.

In my opinion, a good sex life makes a difference in the health of the pelvic region. For example, it exercises the genital, perineal, abdominal, and coccygeus muscles. In addition, sex promotes the circulation of fluids; remember how richly the lesser pelvis is endowed with venous plexuses.

For the most part, physiologists do not think that male orgasm is linked to ejaculation, but instead occurs because of the synchronic and sudden contraction of the muscles of the pelvic floor and the muscular fibers of the seminal colliculus. This is another good reason to stimulate this whole region with physical activity.

Tobacco and Alcohol

Many physicians fail to blame tobacco and alcohol. But do they really know all their ill effects? For example, do they speak of changes in skin, hair, and muscles as signs of tobacco damage? Anyone can usually recognize a smoker immediately by their hair and skin.

Alcohol is a toxin that causes significant vascular problems. Even if alcohol has no direct effect on BPH, its harmful impact on vascular and lymphatic circulation can have an indirect effect.

Venereal Disease

No proven link exists between venereal disease and BPH.

Eating Habits

It is standard procedure that men with BPH are advised to avoid alcohol (especially white wine), spices, chocolate, fat, and red meat. On the other hand, it is recommended that they increase their consumption of vegetables, particularly tomatoes and broccoli, use flaxseed and canola oils, eat flax seeds and papayas, and add a few drop of lemon juice to their drinking water.

Pollution

With pollution it is also difficult to find irrefutable proof of a connection, but serious environmental problems may explain numerous pathologies.

Vertebral Problems

There is no formal evidence that BPH can result from vertebral or coccygeal dysfunction. However the circulatory repercussions imply that they could accelerate and worsen an adenoma process.

Renal Disorders

Although not yet formally demonstrated, it seems that a fairly clear relationship exists between the left kidney and BPH. And by the same reasoning the inverse applies: BPH can cause renal problems.

General Causes

It is advisable that men suffering from BPH avoid a sedentary lifestyle, periods of prolonged sitting, and exposure to cold.

Anesthesia seems to aggravate BPH. Decompensation is often observed after surgery.

Clinical Signs

BPH comes on progressively and silently. Clear clinical signs do not appear until such time as inflammation and fibrosity cause urethral compression. Here are the main signs of BPH:

- Diminished urine stream.
- Dysuria: difficult discharge of urine, initially compensated by increased detrusor muscle contraction. More rarely, there is pain with urination.
- Urinary hesitancy: the patient has the urge to urinate, but no urine emerges for several seconds.
- A weak stream.
- An intermittent stream.
- Abdominal participation: when the patient urinates, he simultaneously contracts his abdominal muscles.
- Manual help: when urinating, the patient compresses his lower abdomen with his free hand.
- Urinary urgency: the sudden desire to void.
- Urinary retention: the patient experiences incomplete emptying of the bladder and must start again several times.
- Diurnal and nocturnal pollakiuria: the frequent passage of small amounts of urine. The patient gets up several times during the night. Because this change develops over time, he thinks it is normal. However, arising more than twice a night to urinate can indicate BPH.
- Bladder distention: the bladder fails to empty completely. Resid-

ual urine stagnates and causes the bladder to distend slightly, with the possible risk of infection or stone formation.

- Detrusor hypertrophy: as the flow of urine is impeded, the detrusor muscle hypertrophies. Very rapidly, diverticula and trabeculae appear.
- Vesicouretic reflux: the bladder weakens with effort. From a state of hypertrophy it shrinks, becomes distended, and loses muscle tone. The junction between the ureter and the bladder becomes dysfunctional, and when the patient strains to void, urine tends to reflux toward the ureter. This creates an open door to infections.
- Renal problems: these vary from simple kidney pain (fairly acute) when urinating to nephritis associated with hydronephrosis.
- Venous stasis: the entire venous system of the lesser pelvis is affected by the mechanical problems discussed above. With periprostatic varicosities one often finds hemorrhoids. The prostatic and periprostatic veins play an important role in intraprostatic pressure. In addition, they protect the prostate from mechanical damage.
- Inguinal hernias can be the result or the cause of male genital problems. The strain of urinating can cause the walls of the inguinal canal to weaken. Remember that inguinal hernias are more frequent in men than in women because the content of the canal is much greater.
- An inguinal hernia can interfere with venous and lymphatic circulation of the genitals and the left kidney.
- Lumbago and sciatica: these are most commonly found of the left side and at night.
- Obstructed bladder: this is an acute retention of urine, is extremely painful, and requires immediate medical attention.

Caution: some medications have iatrogenic effects on the prostate, such as adrenergic stimulants, tranquilizers, nasal drops, antidepressants, antispasmodics, and anesthetics.

Evolution

Left untreated, prostatic adenopathy can create:

- urinary retention
- bladder diverticula
- urinary tract infection
- hematuria
- hydronephrosis
- incontinence
- inguinal hernia
- hemorrhoids
- urinary difficulties
- ejaculatory problems
- lumbago and sciatica
- pelvic pain
- psychological disturbances

Lumbago and Sciatica

Lower-back pain and sciatica are most frequently located on the left side because the left testicular vein empties directly into the left renal vein. By contrast, the venous return from the right testicular flows directly into the vena cava.

In addition to the pain caused by certain activities, prostate-related pain is nocturnal, which is not true of mechanical lower-back pain. With pain of purely mechanical origin, the backache manifests during the night only with a change in position.

Examination

External Palpation

Before any internal examination, evaluate for:

- *Inguinal hernia:* these frequently occur with benign prostatic hypertrophy, as a result of effort during urination.
- *Lymphatic ganglions:* search for inguinal and abdominal ganglions. In the case of adenitis, be very careful; this indicates a probability of infection or tissue invasion.
- Palpation of the *lumbar fossa* and the *kidney* is indispensable in the discovery of possible hydronephrosis and kidney pain. Before manipulating the prostate directly, mobilize the kidneys. This mobilization allows you to take into account any abnormal sensitivity of the kidneys.

Rectal Examination

Rectal examination consists of evaluating the following parameters of the prostate:

- overall size
- contour regularity
- general firmness
- any localized hardness (note: any palpable nodule, induration, or irregularity can be a sign of cancer.)
- elasticity
- anterior-posterior and lateral Mobility
- sensitivity (possible prostatitis)
- absence of the median sulcus
- the urge to urinate on compression

Several more features essential for manual therapy treatment will be explained in detail. Meanwhile, remember that the median sulcus is normally readily palpable. This furrow marks the division of the prostate gland into two ovoid lobes.

Differential Diagnosis Palpation

- A uniform enlargement, clearly defined, painless, firm yet fairly elastic, signifies *benign prostatic hypertrophy.*
- A slightly hardened mass, very painful to the touch and often involving only one lobe, indicates *prostatitis.*
- A sclerosed irregular induration without precise borders is more often than not a sign of *prostate cancer.*

Supplementary Tests

Urinalysis

This is the standard bacteriologic culture test used to diagnose a urinary tract infection or hematuria.

Blood Analysis

Urea and creatinine blood levels indicate a possible renal problem.

PSA Test

PSA stands for prostate-specific antigen. This protein is produced in minute quantities by prostate cells, but is produced in much larger quantities by cancerous cells. There has been an important evolution in the diagnostic value of PSA levels. Today, one rates PSA based on the total PSA. The lower the reported total PSA, the greater the probability of cancer.

Note that not all elevated prostate-specific antigen levels indicate cancer. High PSA levels are observed with:

- BPH (moderate)
- prostate cancer
- acute prostatitis
- urine retention
- rectal examination
- recent ejaculation
- prolonged sitting (cycling, driving, etc.)
- manipulation of the coccyx

Transrectal Ultrasound

Transrectal ultrasound reveals the size and shape of the prostate.

Biopsy

A biopsy is performed using a rectal probe in conjunction with ultrasound. The surgeon takes several tissue samples for study.

Treatments

Medical Treatments

Medical treatments are not within the scope of our practice. However, as our patients frequently talk to us about their medical treatments, it is useful to cite them here.

Plant Extracts

- The African plum tree *(Pygeum africanum):* the skin of this plum has a key active ingredient for the health of the prostate and on the effects of BPH.
- The Florida saw palmetto *(Serenoa repens):* this tree may have a hormone-regulating effect, slowing the development of an adenoma.

Alpha Blockers

These drugs do not target the adenoma but act on the smooth muscles of sphincters and the striated and smooth muscle of the bladder neck and of the urethra. They act on the alpha-adrenergic receptors of the muscle fibers of the entire urogenital system. They are also prescribed for arterial hypertension because of their effect on the arterial vasomotor system.

Hormone Treatment

The objective of hormone treatment is to counter the androgenic stimulation of prostate cancer and BPH. Estrogens are sometimes used, but their side effects are such that this type of treatment is on the verge of being abandoned. Patients have a significant risk of gynecomastia (excessive development of the breast in the male). Several of my patients were so well-developed that they underwent breast-reduction surgery. In addition, they suffer thrombovenous problems.

These treatments are often associated with alpha blockers.

Surgery
Endoscopic Surgery

Endoscopic transurethral prostate resection is common for small adenomas. Shavings of prostatic tissue are removed at the bladder opening. Even when well executed, this technique often has side effects, such as:

- retrograde ejaculation
- urinary incontinence
- impotence (relative or complete)

Impotence

Curiously, most surgeons and authors minimize the risk of impotence. Many patients despair of this problem and are disheartened that it has no solution. When they return to visit their surgeons, they are told they have psychological problems. The erectile nerves run alongside the prostate's lateral borders. The surgical removal of these small nerves results in vascular changes incompatible with an erection. A good surgeon could therefore reduce the risks of impotence.

Retrograde Ejaculation

At the moment of ejaculation, the neck of the bladder closes and the seminal fluid is directed toward the urethra. The prostate rhythmically contracts and the sphincter relaxes suddenly to emit the ejaculation stream. Prostate resection is performed on the bladder neck to restore satisfactory urinary stream. However, the neck remains permanently open, resulting in the ejaculation of semen in a reverse direction, into the urinary bladder.

This event has no physiological effect on the erection or the man's pleasure, surgeons say. Curiously, books devoted to this problem rarely say anything about the pleasure of one's partner at the moment of ejaculation. Sexual pleasure is shared between two partners, and in the case of retrograde ejaculation, both are frustrated. Great progress will be made when the discussion is about true sexuality and not isolated pleasure.

Abdominal Surgery

This type of surgery is reserved for large adenomas. A suprapubic incision is made, and the bladder is opened. This approach entails more or less the same drawbacks as the transurethral option, except the risk of incontinence is greater. Following this type of surgery, ejaculation is retrograde 100 percent of the time.

Other Techniques

Radiotherapy, laser treatment, cryotherapy, thermotherapy, radiation: these techniques are not yet very convincing, and their iatrogenic risks are not negligible.

Note that following radiation therapy, internal prostate manipulation is to be done with the utmost caution. The periprostatic tissues are all irritated and become fragile. The greatest risk is hemorrhage because of the acquired weakness of the arterial and venous walls.

Advice and Precautions

Be Physically Active

Physical activity mobilizes the tissues, prevents venous stasis, and stimulates all major functions.

Empty the Bladder Completely

It is important that the patient void the bladder regularly without waiting until the last moment. An overfull bladder promotes prostatic and venous congestion. The bladder muscle thickens, and this invites diverticula.

Avoid Long Periods of Sitting or Lying Down

Prolonged sitting is specifically to be avoided as it causes lymph and blood stasis, leading to congestion of the prostate and the bladder. This is a problem for those who, because of their profession, must remain seated for long periods.

Cycling can also promote problems; in my opinion, however, it is more the urethra that is irritated in this activity. Such mechanical urethritis can cause irritation and congestion of the prostate.

Follow a Good Diet

Be careful with spices, alcohol (particularly white wine), chocolate, overly acidic food, red meat, and fats. Patients should be advised to consume more vegetables and regularly to sip small quantities of water with a few drops of lemon added.

Note: Whenever there is the slightest doubt, always take the advice of a specialist. An excellent manual prostate exam is certainly not sufficient to make sure there is nothing suspicious or to be concerned about.

Prostate Cancer

At present it is rare for an osteopath or manual therapist to be the first to discover prostate cancer. While it is not yet systematic, testing PSA levels is becoming standard. It is more and more common for general practitioners to perform rectal exams on their patients, to the extent that many patients arrive for manual therapy consultation after receiving medical advice. This is a very good thing.

Nevertheless, an osteopath or manual therapist must be familiar with the characteristic features of prostate cancer. As it happens, frequent falls on the coccyx inevitably lead to the common practice of rectal examination. During examination of the coccyx, it is important that the osteopath or manual therapist verify that everything is normal with the prostate, referring to a urologist any patient that presents with questionable findings.

Definition

Prostate cancer is an adenoma carcinoma. Seventy percent develop in the peripheral zone most accessible to rectal examination; 15–20 percent are found in the central zone, and 10–15 percent are located in the transitional area of the prostate.

The cancer can spread across the prostatic capsule toward the base of the seminal vesicles and toward the lymphatic ganglions. More rarely, it spreads to the bladder neck and the lower ureters. The younger the patient, the more rapidly the cancer advances.

Frequency

In France, prostate cancer is the second leading cause of death in men after lung and colon cancers. Due to earlier detection and the aging of the population, more and more prostate cancers are discovered. During autopsies it is very common to find cancers of the prostate that the patient, having died of another cause, was unaware of.

For some years now, prostate cancers have been found by rheumatologists. Patients seek consultation for lower-back pain that is extremely painful and unresponsive to treatment. It is common for prostate cancer to metastasize to the bones.

Examinations
Digital Rectal Exam

This examination is primary, simple, painless, and harmless. It detects contour irregularities but does not provide information as to the quality or seriousness of an adenoma. During the rectal exam, contour anomalies and bulk are signs that define the side concerned.

You must also evaluate the periprostatic area for possible extraprostatic tissue proliferation, and palpate the seminal vesicles.

Urologists confirm that a hardened and circumscribed surface on the contour of the prostate is cancerous 50 percent of the time.

It should be reiterated that during a rectal exam carried out on a patient with a sacrococcygeal problem, osteopaths and manual therapists can certainly be the first to discover a prostate anomaly. Prostate cancer is found most commonly in the caudal prostate. The cranial part, even when hypertrophic, does not become cancerous.

PSA Levels

Most men, even without specific urinary complaints, routinely undergo systematic cancer detection through a test of PSA levels. A PSA rate lower than normal may be suspicious if it was much lower the previous year, and if the relationship between free PSA and total PSA has decreased from one year to the next.

Note: The diagnosis of cancer of the prostate is uniquely based on anatomic pathology.

Symptomatology

At the beginning, there is no specific symptomatology to prostate cancer. The signs are the same as those described above for benign prostatic hypertrophy. On the other hand, if the cancer is already well advanced, the patient can suffer characteristic painful vertebrae.

Painful Vertebrae

With men over age fifty who complain of lower-back pain or sciatica without apparent mechanical cause, it is useful to ask several important questions:

- Does the pain occur at night?
- Is it triggered by physical activity or poor body position?
- Does it occur frequently while at rest?
- Is it aggravated by physical activity?
- Is it worse with a full bladder?
- Is it relieved after urinating?
- Is it soothed by assuming a more comfortable position?

Recall that in the case of lower-back pain of mechanical origin, rest relieves the discomfort. The pain improves after a good night's sleep. It is aggravated by physical activity and soothed by shifting to a more comfortable body position.

Sometimes the problem is complex. A patient with asymptomatic prostate cancer can, after a fall or during intense physical activity, suddenly experience lumbosacral pain. During a consultation he may well focus your attention on the recent event to the point that you may forget to be vigilant.

Metastasis

In medicine, the basic treatment for cancer that metastasizes to the bone is blocking androgens, theoretically to slow tumor growth. Truth be told, there is no real treatment for metastasis, and the patient suffers enormously. I have heard courageous patients howl with pain. There is not much that manual therapy can do for them. Happily, there has been great progress made in opiate medications; administered in proper dosages, morphine eases intolerable pain.

Risk Factors

Genetic Influence

If a man's father or brother has had prostate cancer, his risk of developing it doubles or even triples. General familial risk (grandfather, uncle) is the same whether on the mother's side or the father's side.

Ethnic Factors

African Americans have an elevated risk of prostate cancer. Asians in the United States have a lower rate of prostate cancer than do African Americans, but they are at higher risk than Asians living in Asia. This disparity suggests that other factors are at play.

Dietary Considerations

Food certainly plays a role: excessive consumption of red meat and fats is harmful. Fats can convert into androgens, which may explain their effect on cancer. As with BPH, even if tobacco and alcohol have not been formally identified as causing prostate changes, it makes good sense to avoid them. Suggest to patients that they consume as many vegetables as possible, especially tomatoes, broccoli, and soy products. Vitamin supplements are recommended, particularly vitamins D and E. Some people advise taking trace elements such as selenium and zinc.

Prostatitis

The prostate is a gland that can become inflamed. Infections sometime lie dormant, and episodes recur over the years. There is a big difference between acute and chronic prostatitis.

Acute Prostatitis
Clinical Signs

Acute prostatitis is easy to diagnose. The principal signs are the following:

- Fatigue: the patient experiences sudden fatigue, literally being drained of all energy. With BPH, by contrast, no particular fatigue is noticed.
- Fever: temperature rises rapidly to 102–104 degrees Fahrenheit (39–40 degrees C).
- Urinary tract infection
- Hematuria
- Burning urination
- Considerable abdominal-pelvic pain
- Genital pain

Examinations
Rectal Exam

The prostate is extremely tender and painful. The quality of the pain is so intense that there can be no doubt as to the cause.

Urinalysis

Urinalysis reveals bacterial causes of infection. In acute prostatitis, often *Escherichia coli* (colibacillosis) is found, and less frequently, chlamydia and mycoplasma are detected.

PSA Markers

The PSA test is useless, as irritation and inflammation of the prostate increases PSA levels considerably.

Causes

- Sexually transmitted diseases are most often implicated in young patients. Usually chlamydia and mycoplasma are found. These bacteria are not always easy to detect through urinalysis. The physician must sometimes ask for a urethral swab or a sperm culture.
- Adenoma: this is sometimes a predisposing factor because of the risk of infection it induces.
- Surgery: catheterization following transurethral prostatectomy carries the risk of infection. Patients are often given prophylactic antibiotics to avoid infection.

Treatment

Manual therapy is never appropriate with acute prostatitis. There would be serious risk of spreading the infection. Treatment consists of antibiotics and fluids. Ask the patient to sip small quantities of water at frequent intervals and to avoid ingesting too many animal proteins.

Chronic Prostatitis

There are more candidates for this syndrome in men around the age of fifty. This is a stealthy infection that often manifests in cycles. Sometimes the infection can return years after the previous episode.

Clinical Signs

- Apyrexia: unlike with acute prostatitis, there is no fever.
- Urinary problems:
  - dysuria
  - pollakiuria

- burning urination
- urethral discharge
- pyuria

- Pelvic pain:
  - perivesical
  - penile
  - anal
  - ejaculatory

Rectal Exam

The prostate is often enlarged, painful, and hardened with irregular and nodular contours; sometimes this is suggestive of cancer.

Causes

- Infection: germs are very difficult to identify. Chlamydia and mycoplasma are often involved.
  - urinary tract infection

Predisposing Factors

- stress
- hypoactivity
- poor diet

Associated Problems

In addition to urinary problems, chronic prostatitis can entail:

- *Sterility:* on top of painful symptoms, chronic prostatitis can render a man infertile. It is important to remember that the infection can persist for years, often with no symptoms.

- *Hepatic problems:* one of my patients consulted me regularly for chronic digestive problems whose signs appeared to be a liver problem. The biological analysis tests were normal. One day he telephoned to ask what he should do about urethral discharge. I advised that his doctor order a detailed urinalysis; it revealed a chlamydia infection, which was treated with antibiotics. What is remarkable in this story is that the patient had no other digestive problems. One of the liver's important functions is to help with the elimination of microorganisms and their consequences. It seemed in this case that the liver had itself fallen victim to chlamydia.

- *Relative impotence:* often impotence is not complete but involves a weak or average erection. It manifests in episodes and may be explained by psychological problems. As one patient put it, "It is not easy to accept that your genital organs betray you, and that in taking pleasure they give you nothing but problems."

- *Lumbago:* this arises spontaneously for no apparent reason. Chronic prostatitis irritates the hypogastric plexus, which can cause spasming of the perineal muscles. The resulting venous stasis eventually produces congestion of the epidural veins. This is, of course, only one of several possible explanations. It is also known that the fasciae of the lesser pelvis become tense and can therefore unbalance the reciprocal lumbar myofascial tensions.

Prognosis

Chronic prostatitis can develop over months or even years. The patient is often dispirited by the multiple recurrences, made all the more insidious because between bouts there are no symptoms.

Implications for Manual Therapy

While manual therapy is contraindicated in cases of acute prostatitis, it can be helpful when the signs of infection are not present. The role of the practitioner is to reduce fibrosity in the tissues around the urethra and to restore the prostate to its normal condition of firmness.

Chapter 4

The Manual Approach

Benign Prostatic Hypertrophy, the Seminal Vesicles, and the Periprostatic Tissues

General

Preliminary Conditions

When a practitioner takes on a patient for benign prostatic hypertrophy (BPH), it is preferable that he first consults a physician or a urologist for an objective diagnosis. The situation should never arise where a case of presumed BPH is taken on when in fact the problem is cancer.

Concept of the Global Lesion

This concept clearly asserts that each part of the body is important and indispensable to the whole. The osteopath or manual therapist, being a globalist mechanic, does not have the right to declare that he or she does not do internal manipulation out of personal preference when it falls within the scope of practice. It is not for us to decide which parts of the body are important to treat; only the tissues know. This book discusses patients and not a therapist's personal discomfort. It is possible to change the quality of a patient's life by helping him avoid prostate surgery and its considerable attendant risks, and it is simply not feasible to manipulate the prostatic urethra except via the internal route.

Similarly, in the case of women, what viable reason would persuade a therapist not to manipulate the uterus and its attachments in an infertile woman? To help a woman conceive a child is one of the noblest missions in life. From the moment an osteopath or manual therapist accepts to help the body of a patient in its totality, he or she takes a big step toward respecting people and their suffering. This is the proof that the patient matters more than his own concerns. In my opinion, an osteopath or manual therapist who practices internal manipulation understands that he must do everything possible to help the patient.

Manual Therapy as a First Resort

As discussed above, surgical treatments or medications for BPH carry risks for the patient. Manual therapy, which has no iatrogenic effects, is a better first try.

In view of the importance of the symptoms, patients are asked to come for three or four consultations spaced three weeks to one month apart. After these sessions, they are advised to return in three to four months so that the results can be judged. If there is no change, it is preferable to abandon manual therapy. It is useful to set a limit on treatment.

Purpose of Manual Therapy

Important: the goal is not to reduce the volume of the adenoma but to intervene with the consequences of its enlargement. Manipulation has little impact on the size of the prostate, but it affects the functional problems caused by an enlarged prostate.

Objective Tests

At present, many osteopaths and manual therapists duplicate objective exams of patients to establish proof of the effectiveness of manual therapy. I include myself in this category. Today there are a multitude of theses developed with the eventual goal that by force of statistics, manual therapy will be seen objectively rather than subjectively.

In the case of the prostate, the only objective test would be to show that after three or four manipulations, the size of the prostate clearly diminishes by an accurate and clear measure. However, urologists are in agreement that it is not the size of the prostate that matters. An enlarged prostate can become enlarged in the dorsal direction, that is to say projecting toward the rectum, without creating any particular disturbance.

Excellent results have been achieved on prostates that have not altered in dimension but that have recovered good Mobility and condition. The urethra became less compressed, and urinary symptoms were reduced and sometimes even disappeared.

Purpose of Prostate Manipulation

Here are the various parameters that osteopaths and manual therapists seek to affect.

Mechanical Goal

Manipulation of the prostate influences:

- Mobility
- Motility
- hardness

- consistency
- extensibility
- elasticity
- intraprostatic pressure
- extraprostatic pressure
- the vas deferens
- the ejaculatory ducts

Neurological Goal

The prostatic and periprostatic tissues, notably Denonvilliers's fascia, are rich in smooth muscle fibers. They react to manual manipulation because their musculoligamentous system is highly proprioceptive. The prostate also reacts more easily and intensely than do simple supportive tissues. Manipulation works either:

- directly on the nervous system of the prostate, by way of the hypogastric plexus and nerve fibers issuing from the lumbar and sacral plexus.
- indirectly through the propagation of proprioceptive nerve impulses that relay to the cerebellum and thalamus.

Vascular Goal

It is thought that particularly at the level of the rich venous framework surrounding the prostate, manual manipulation plays a role:

- directly by mobilizing the venous contents.
- indirectly through the nervous system of the venous walls.

Lymphatic Goal

The prostate is surrounded by a rich lymphatic network, especially well developed at the posterior part, accessible by the finger. By improving lymphatic circulation it seems logical that manipulation can benefit the gland's immune system.

Hormonal Goal

The experiments that I have conducted with my friend and colleague Alain Croibier, DO, show that precise manipulation of one part of the body systematically activates the thalamus. This event then triggers other central reactions, whether they be limbic, hypothalamic, or some other reaction. Although there is no formal proof as of yet, we believe that prostate manipulation has a central hormonal effect. The gynecologists Lecomte and Lansac have demonstrated that simple mobilization of the neck of the uterus causes an increase in prostaglandin levels; why not in the prostate?

Prostaglandins

Sperm has a large concentration of prostaglandins. Physiologists think that prostaglandins induce relaxation of the uterus neck to facilitate the penetration of spermatozoa. At the same time, these hormones may promote contractions of the body of the uterus in order to accelerate the transit of sperm as far as the junction of the uterus and uterine tubes.

Any organ that is congested, sensitive, somewhat immobile, or indurated cannot have beneficial effects on the organism. Restoring the organ to its proper condition improves homeostasis and stimulates the larger functions.

Functional Goal

Internal prostate manipulation also affects the ureter, the ejaculator ducts, the ductus deferens, and the seminal vesicles. This is because the stretching of any tube improves its peristalsis and lumen. The intention is also to stimulate the precise areas in the brain that corresponds to the prostate. Every organ is represented by a specific area in the brain. Mobilizing the prostate stimulates its cerebral counterpart, and in this way a retroactive benefit is achieved.

Effects of Manipulation
Effects on Urinary Problems

Essentially, urinary problems are where the effects of manipulation are most easily recognized. A man who had to get up three or four times during the night to urinate before treatment, and who now gets up just once, knows that you have helped.

Effects on Infections

Men are more commonly treated for mechanical rather than infectious urinary problems. While I have less experience with the latter, I have nevertheless been able to reduce acute episodes of chronic prostatitis significantly.

Effects on Fertility

For fertility there is no formal evidence either, but many patients have assured me that after manipulating their prostates, ejaculations became easier. In fact, they noticed mechanical and quantitative improvement. Several patients are convinced that the value of their spermiogram has improved thanks to treatment. However, I prefer to remain cautious in regard to such assertions. It is known that spermatogenesis takes about seventy-four days, and the transport of the spermatozoa requires twelve to fourteen days. Thus one would have to wait three months to retake a meaningful spermiogram, without the intervention of other factors, to prove the beneficial effect of manual therapy.

Effects on Impotence

There are so many physical and psychological factors associated with impotence that it is difficult to be clear about it. Experience has shown numerous times that the best results are achieved when lumbosacral manipulation is combined with prostate treatment. That is to say, patients suffering from both vertebral and prostate problems show the best results from manipulation. The spinal segments responsible for erections are S2 to S4 and T12 to L2. In my experience it is upper lumbar manipulation in particular that has an effect on impotence.

Very often men broach the subject of impotence with great difficulty. The first positive results I obtained with the prostate were accomplished without discussing erectile problems. During follow-up consultations patients said things like, "My back is much better, and everything else is too." I asked, "What do you mean by 'everything else'?" The response was, "You know very well what I'm trying to say." The practitioner must know how to interpret such messages.

Patient Information

I don't believe in the practice of saying to patients, "You've come to the right place; you'll see that everything is going to be fine." I explain to patients that more than from the interview, my hands will discover what is important to treat. The more prostatic and periprostatic fixations are found, the more manual manipulation techniques succeed. Patients are asked to have three or four sessions and to observe the results themselves.

Contraindications

Certain signs or symptoms are cause for extreme caution. Manipulation should be postponed, or the advice of a specialist should be sought if the patient is experiencing:

- fever
- adenitis, adenolymphitis
- intense pelvic pain, spontaneous or provoked
- pyuria
- hematuria
- significant weight loss
- obsession with genital matters
- nocturnal lumbosacral pain

Precautions

Be careful with patients who have or have had:

- abdominal pelvic radiotherapy; even if it was not specifically over the genitals, there is a risk of hemorrhage due to vascular fragility.
- anticoagulant medication
- cortisone

Follow these precautions:

- Ask the patient to empty his bladder before treatment.
- Warn him that he may feel the urge to urinate during manipulation, but that this is more likely just a strong impulse rather than a real necessity.
- It is possible that the presence of a finger in the rectum may cause an impulse to defecate. Reassure him that again, this is more an urge than a real risk.

- Place several absorbent cloths on the table to provide further reassurance. In the hundreds of cases I have treated, only one patient began urinating during prostate manipulation.
- Most of the time patients think they have lost a bit of urine when actually nothing happened. This feeling is due to the stimulation of the hypogastric plexus and the pudendal nerves.
- Inform the patient that following treatment he may lose a few drops of urine. Ask him to check whether they are drops of pus, in which case a more thorough investigation is warranted.

External Tests

True testing of the prostate, seminal vesicles, and periprostatic tissues is done internally. There are nevertheless some external tests that can give clues to a prostate problem. In my opinion, the most revealing evaluation is abdominopelvic Listening.

Abdominopelvic Listening Test

This is a general pelvic evaluation. The patient lies face-up with legs extended and arms lying alongside the body. Place the palm of your dominant hand against the pubic symphysis, index finger along the midline pointing toward the umbilicus. Allow your hand to be passively moved where it is attracted.

Be careful: it is the movement of the palm—not the fingers—that indicates the location of the problem. For example, when the palm goes left, the fingers turn toward the right; the problem is clearly located on the left.

Differential Manual Evaluation

The Prostate

The palm makes a cubital rotation whereby the pisiform comes to rest slightly to the left of the umbilicopubic line, against the pubis, and then is drawn somewhat deeper (fig. 4.1). Note that Listening is done the same way as for the neck of the uterus.

The Sigmoid

It is possible to confuse sigmoid Listening for that of the prostate. For the sigmoid, the palm remains flat; it glides laterally over a large surface before making a slight cubital rotation. The fact that the palm is drawn less deeply is what differentiates sigmoid Listening from prostate Listening.

The Bladder

When there is a problem in the caudal part of the bladder, the palm is immediately drawn dorsally. It deviates slightly from the umbilicopubic line and above all does not come against the pubis.

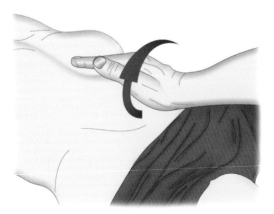

Figure 4.1. Testing the prostate using abdominopelvic Listening.

The Seminal Vesicles

It is difficult to distinguish these structures from the prostate. The pisiform makes a cubital rotation but without coming to rest against the pubis.

External Manipulation

Prostate manipulation is performed internally or externally. Internal techniques are the most effective. Nevertheless, before embarking on internal manipulation, it is a good idea to treat neighboring organs and other tissues that influence the prostate. External manipulation ensures that conditions are optimal for successful internal work. The value of treating specific organs in conjunction with helping the prostate is described below. Their manipulation will not be described in detail, however; you can refer to other texts dedicated to the subject.

The Kidneys

The left kidney is of particular importance to the prostate. This is because of its venous system, which is dependent on the left testicular (spermatic) vein (figs. 4.2 and 4.3). The right testicular vein empties directly into the inferior vena cava, whereas the left testicular vein opens into the left renal vein.

All genital problems have repercussions for the left kidney and vice versa. The testicular veins form an important convoluted network called the pampiniform plexus. Venous stasis can cause varicosities in the spermatic cords and the testicles, setting up the conditions for hydroceles or low sperm count.

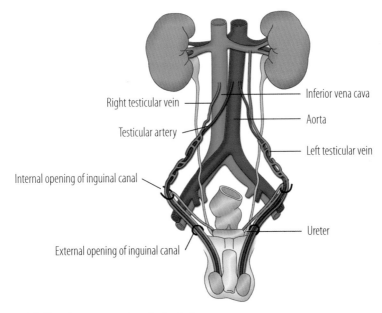

Right testicular vein

Testicular artery

Internal opening of inguinal canal

External opening of inguinal canal

Inferior vena cava

Aorta

Left testicular vein

Ureter

Figure 4.2. Renal nervous system (adapted from Helga Fritsch and Wolfgang Kuhnel).

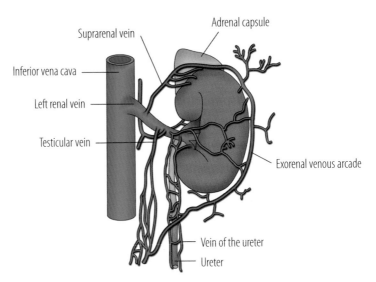

Suprarenal vein

Adrenal capsule

Inferior vena cava

Left renal vein

Testicular vein

Exorenal venous arcade

Vein of the ureter

Ureter

Figure 4.3. Left renal venous system (adapted from Testut).

Pelvicotrochanter Muscles

Of interest here are the pyramidalis, superior gemellus, obturator internus, inferior gemellus, and quadratus femoris muscles (fig. 4.4). These muscles do not act directly on the prostate, but by their actions contribute to the creation of pressure dynamics in the lesser pelvis, which assists vascular and lymphatic circulation.

My esteemed colleagues Didier Prat and the late Louis Rommeveaux have always delighted in emphasizing the importance that the coxofemoral joint plays and its effect on the bladder. This particular joint action also exerts itself on the prostate and the seminal vesicles by providing a natural and indispensable physiological pumping action.

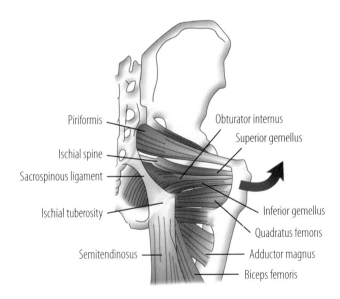

Figure 4.4. Pelvicotrochanter muscles.

Technique

The patient lies face-up with the lower extremities flexed (fig. 4.5). The index and middle finger of the proximal hand are placed against the medial part of the trochanter in the direction of the trochanteric fossa. The distal hand encompasses the bent knee to bring the hip into flexion. The muscles and fascia are relaxed in this position, so take advantage of this to securely make contact toward the trochanter. Allow the fingers to move to where the Listening takes them. Mobilize the lower extremity into abduction-external rotation, then into extension-adduction, and progressively into internal rotation. Throughout the movement, continue to maintain a lateral pull on the greater trochanter.

This is a powerful and sometimes painful maneuver at the beginning as the muscles naturally spasm and are tense. This mobilization technique will stretch and stimulate all of contents of the lesser pelvis, which is especially beneficial to the venous and lymphatic systems and the pelvic organs.

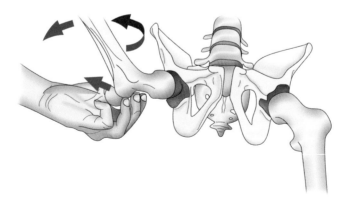

Figure 4.5. Technique for the pelvicotrochanteric muscles.

Sacrosciatic Ligaments

The effects of these ligaments on the lesser pelvis are comparable to those of the pelvicotrochanteric muscles. In addition, they form a liaison between the legs and the pelvis by way of the biceps femoris and hamstrings muscles.

Technique

The patient is in the same position as for the muscles of the hip and thigh above (figs. 4.6 and 4.7). Contact the ischial tuberosity with the fingers of your proximal hand. First, bring the ipsilateral lower extremity into flexion-abduction and external rotation. This will

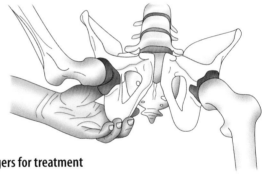

Figure 4.6. Position of the fingers for treatment of the sacrosciatic ligaments.

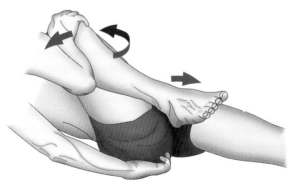

Figure 4.7. Sacrospinous ligament technique.
1: rotation. 2: extension.

allow you better to place your fingers against the proximal part of the ischial tuberosity. Next, bring the lower extremity into adduction-extension while drawing the ischial tuberosity laterally. At the end of the movement, bring the leg into internal rotation. These bands are vestigial muscles that gradually transformed over time into ligaments. They have an important reflexogenic effect on all the organs of the lesser pelvis.

In manual therapy the effect sought is not stretching but rather a proprioceptive effect.

Levator Ani and Perineum

The prostate and the urethra are closely connected to the levator ani muscles and to the perineal structures. These muscles help to balance pressure exerted by the abdomen, and by this means they influence vascular and lymphatic function. They can be manipulated using the ischial spine as the intermediary.

Ischial Spine

The ischial spine (fig. 4.8) is the meeting point of all the key muscles and aponeuroses of the lesser pelvis. It is a strategic location for manipulation in order to affect:

- the levator ani muscle
- the sacrospinous ligament
- the iliococcygeus muscle
- the piriformis muscle
- the superior gemellus muscle
- the obturator internus muscle
- the tendinous arch

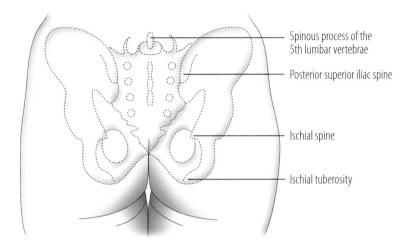

Spinous process of the
5th lumbar vertebrae

Posterior superior iliac spine

Ischial spine

Ischial tuberosity

Figure 4.8. Ischial spine.

Technique

With the patient lying face-up, flex the homolateral knee and ischial spine (fig. 4.9). Stand on the same side. Support the anterior surface of the knee with your distal hand. Place the index and middle fingers of your proximal hand on the medial aspect of the ischial spine. To reach the ischial spine, first locate the ischial tuberosity, then glide you fingers in a cranial and slightly medial direction until you meet it. The ischial spine is situated about four finger-widths from the ischial tuberosity. With your distal hand, bring the knee into flexion and a slight abduction, which will allow you more secure contact against the medial part of the ischial spine. Bring the knee initially into extension-abduction and external rotation while drawing the ischial spine laterally. At the end of extension, bring the lower extremity into internal rotation of the knee, without releasing your lateral traction on the ischial spine.

Figure 4.9. Finger placement for the ischial spine technique.

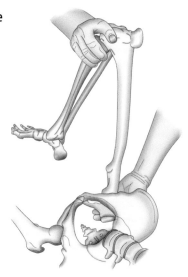

Lumbosacral Plexus

Here a similar technique is applied as for the ischial spine. The only difference consists of directing the fingers of your proximal hand in a cranial direction toward the greater sciatic foramen, where the cranial part of the sacral plexus is located (fig. 4.10). Accordingly, place

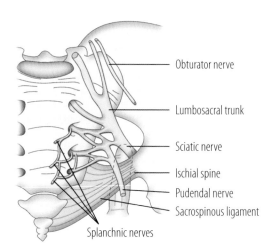

Obturator nerve

Lumbosacral trunk

Sciatic nerve

Ischial spine

Pudendal nerve

Sacrospinous ligament

Splanchnic nerves

Figure 4.10. Manipulation of the lumbosacral plexus.

your finger on the cranial part of the ischial spine and direct it in a cranial direction. As in the ischial spine technique, the distal hand mobilizes the knee and the lower extremity, initially into flexion-abduction and external rotation and then into extension-adduction and internal rotation. The finger in the sciatic foramen tries to feel a more sensitive area to stretch. If no sensitivity is found, the finger follows the Local Listening.

The Bladder

The prostate has quasidirect links with the bladder. Furthermore, the bladder's system of attachments often exchanges fibers with the prostate. The urachus, pubovesical ligaments, pubourethral ligaments, and the sacro-recto-genito-pubic aponeurosis all have a fairly direct action on the prostate.

You can refer to texts devoted to the bladder, but below is a technique that unites the bladder with the sacrum. This technique is inspired by a maneuver developed by my excellent colleague and friend Bernard Lignier. In addition to all the techniques concerning the urachus, the medial umbilical ligaments, the pubovesical ligaments, and the wings of the bladder, the following vesico-prostato-sacral technique is used.

Vesico-prostato-sacral Technique

With the patient lying face-up, place the palm of your ventral hand against the superior border of the pubic symphysis, your fingers pointing toward the pubis. Your dorsal hand is placed on the sacrum between S2 and S4. Carry out a pumping action between your two hands, in effect compressing and decompressing the vesicosacral region. To accentuate the musculoaponeurotic traction effect, draw the palm of the abdominal hand in a cranial direction and move the sacral contact caudal. First, compress the tissue, and then follow with the traction procedure.

Lumbar Spine

Can a fixation in the lumbar spine cause susceptibility to prostatic adenoma? This is a difficult question to answer. It is known that a vertebral restriction has consequences for fluid circulation in the lesser pelvis, especially in the venous system. In my view, even if it is not a direct cause, it is a good idea to manipulate the lumbar vertebral column when there is a strong fixation. Leaving a spinal fixation unresolved reduces the chances of overall success.

Primary or Secondary

Manual therapists and osteopaths have become accustomed to manipulating the visceral system before adjusting the vertebral column. If the spine is secondary to a prostate fixation, it will self-correct immediately following mobilization of the prostate.

L1, L2, and L3 are the lumbar vertebrae that are most commonly found fixated in conjunction with prostate fixation. Most of the time, the secondary lumbar fixation is restricted to one side. That is to say, only one interapophyseal articulation is blocked. Manipulation of a vertebral segment restricted on only one side is not indicated; it is almost always a compensation. In removing the compensation, the patient risks developing very acute sciatica in the days or weeks following such a spinal adjustment.

Rectal Examination

The precautions to take and the advice to follow have been reviewed above. One thing is very important: you must explain clearly and soberly what you are going to do. *Any discomfort here comes from the therapist and not from the patient.* This kind of squeamishness is particularly unacceptable considering all the problems that a patient endures with BPH. The patient fervently hopes that you are going to help him and perhaps even allow him to avoid surgery. He is counting on you and therefore gives you carte blanche.

Be sober and brief in your explanation; an overly lengthy description is a sign of reluctance to proceed to the actual technique. The patient will sense this immediately and little by little lose his confidence in you.

Is It Painful?

This question is practically automatic with patients. Most often they have been burned by an aggressive rectal technique undertaken for a coccygeal problem or prostate examination. No, rectal palpation is not painful, as long as you respect the tensions in the tissues and you personally are at ease. The best answer is to say that it may not be pleasant but it is not painful either.

Precautions

If you feel small amounts of fecal matter in the rectal ampulla, delicately reposition them in the cranial direction to avoid any annoyance for the patient, notably a strong urge to defecate. With this type of impulse, all the muscles of the lesser pelvis are in a defensive position and render manipulation difficult.

Position

It is far preferable to have the patient lying on his stomach rather than on his back or on all fours. The patient feels more protected and less exposed. Ask the patient to lie flat on his stomach with his briefs on. Once he is on the table you can lower his underwear.

Technique

With a small amount of lubricant on your gloved index finger, place your finger pad face up in the direction of the ventral surface of the sacrum. Lay the palm of your external hand directly on the sacrum and gradually increase the pressure so that the patient's attention becomes fixed on the sacrum. Position your index finger at the entrance of the anal sphincter and penetrate very slightly. As a rule, the patient tenses instantaneously. Do not tell him to relax. On the contrary, ask him to strongly contract his buttock muscles and then relax them. At the moment of relaxation, you can glide your finger slowly inward. Continue in this manner several times. Once the first phalanx has penetrated, the rest of the index finger follows very easily. Direct your index finger along a 40 degree angle, approximately in line with the axis of the body. The finger pad faces the sacrum, and at this stage it is possible to check for possible hemorrhoids.

Hemorrhoids

When you direct the finger pad against the anterior surface of the sacrum, you will feel a slight resistance under your finger. The feeling is comparable to damp hair. If you feel this, it is likely hemorrhoids. Check to make sure that compressing them against the sacrum or stretching them in a ventral direction causes no pain. There may be slight indurations on these interlaced filaments. This indicates microvaricosities.

Local Hemorrhoid Treatment

Stretch the hemorrhoids in a ventral direction by moving the index finger into extension. Do this several times, modifying the direction of your finger slightly each time. This technique decongests the dilated veins and helps the venous circulation of the hemorrhoidal plexus. Occasionally the hemorrhoidal veins spiral against each other and form a thrombus, which is very painful.

This treatment is very effective in acute hemorrhoid attacks. It takes away the pain almost instantaneously. Following treatment the patient is advised to have several sitz baths in water made very cold by placing ice cubes in it. Also, the simple act of placing an ice cube in the rectum is often enough to eliminate the pain.

Implications for the Prostate

The prostate is surrounded by a rich endowment of venous plexus that can become varicosed. Such varicosities often accompany other varicosities located in the organs of the lesser pelvis, notably the rectum. Improving rectal venous circulation relieves the prostate by making it more functional and strengthening its immune defenses.

Note: along with any local hemorrhoid treatment, always remember to provide counsel concerning the optimal function of the liver: avoid alcohol, chocolate, and heated fats, for example.

Periprostatic Tissues

Sacrococcygeal Test

During rectal palpation, it is imperative to check the sacrococcygeal articulation. A fixation of this junction can produce numerous nociceptive effects on the body. It can interfere with arteriovenous circulation and create continuous spasms of the urogenital muscles as well as of the smooth muscle fibers of their system of attachment.

Technique

Place the index finger in the rectum against the ventral surface of the coccyx and sacrum, moving little by little as far as possible in a cranial direction. The thumb of the same hand is placed on the external surface of the dorsal coccyx and the caudal end of the sacrum. The two fingers move the sacrococcygeal joint into flexion to evaluate the anterior sacrococcygeal ligaments, and into extension to test the posterior sacrococcygeal ligaments. Also evaluate the elasticity of the lateral sacrococcygeal fibers by mobilizing the coccyx several times. A Mobility restriction is almost always accompanied by a fixation of the homolateral sacrospinous ligament. As a rule, only the anterior coccygeal ligament fixation is painful on mobilization. Being the most reflexogenic, this fixation is well worth seeking out.

Sacrospinous and Sacrotuberous Ligaments

These powerful ligaments are the vestiges of tail muscles. The ancients referred to them as *agitator caudae,* and they mobilized the tail laterally. Sometimes discovered in them are smooth muscle fibers arising from the coccygeal muscle.

In my experience, the sacrospinous ligament is the most reflexogenic and receptive to manipulation. However, the fibers of these two structures are so very intermingled that it is difficult to separate them on the mechanical and reflexogenic planes. The sacrospinous and sacrotuberous ligaments are virtually always restricted in the case of a sacrococcygeal fixation or with problems of the homolateral lower extremity. In terms of the fixation, it is also common to find a visceral problem:

- On the left: the sigmoid, rectum, descending colon, left kidney, or the prostate.
- On the right: the right kidney, the cecum, or the descending colon.

Test

The rectal finger is directed caudal and lateral, without attempting to go dorsally at the start (fig. 4.11). Then lift the finger in a dorsal direction, and you will feel the flat hard cord of the sacrotuberous ligament. The thumb of the external hand goes to meet the rectal finger to get a good sense of the distensibility of this ligament. Always com-

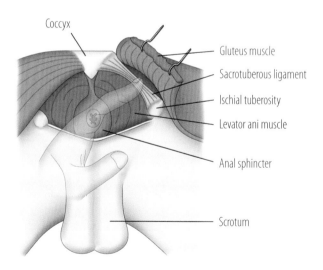

Coccyx
Gluteus muscle
Sacrotuberous ligament
Ischial tuberosity
Levator ani muscle
Anal sphincter
Scrotum

Figure 4.11. Test of the sacrotuberous ligament by the internal route.

pare both sides. A fixation manifests as a fibrous condition with more limited extensibility.

A Mobility restriction of the sacrospinous ligament is always accompanied by a fixation of the sacrotuberous ligament, especially its inferior part. The sacrospinous ligament attaches to the sciatic spine, which is a key point of attachment for the muscles and ligaments of the pelvis. It is advantageous to test the other structures that attach to this bone and the neighboring structures, for example the piriformis, coccygeus, and obturator internus muscles.

Treatment
Internal Route

The intrarectal finger comes up against the sacrospinous ligament while the external thumb goes to the same place externally (fig. 4.12). The two carry out a simultaneous Induction technique; in general,

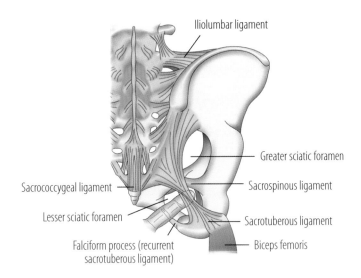

Iliolumbar ligament

Greater sciatic foramen

Sacrospinous ligament

Sacrotuberous ligament

Biceps femoris

Sacrococcygeal ligament

Lesser sciatic foramen

Falciform process (recurrent sacrotuberous ligament)

Figure 4.12. Internal manipulation of the sacrospinous and sacrotuberous ligaments.

five to six times suffices. It is important to feel an improvement in distensibility. As this ligament has some muscular fibers, it responds very well to Induction. Its release brings relaxation to the sacrotuberous ligament.

External Route

The patient is lying down on his side, the side opposite the ligaments to be treated. This is the classic lumbar roll position. Place the palm of your hand or back of the forearm against the ischial tuberosity. Draw the tuberosity cranially and laterally to engage the ligaments. The goal is to put the ligaments into maximum stretch.

Advice to the Patient

Ask the patient to stretch these ligaments himself. He does this by grasping his knee with both hands and bringing it toward the opposite shoulder. This can be accomplished lying down or in a seated position.

Sacral Periosteum

Some falls on the coccyx or sacrum cause intracartilaginous or intraosseous lesions to form. These manifest as small, sensitive transverse periosteal folds located on the anterior surface of the sacrum. These can show up on the natural transverse ridges of the anterior sacrum, corresponding to the vestiges of the five sacral vertebral joints, or just beside them (fig. 4.13).

These sensitive folds have an important reflexogenic effect, to the extent that they can be the origin of pelvic visceral spasm and ejaculatory dysfunction.

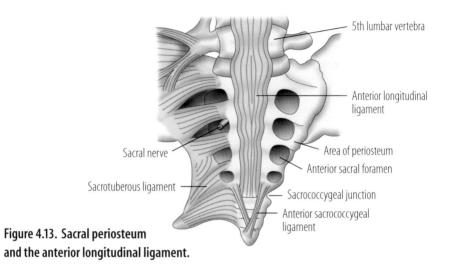

5th lumbar vertebra

Anterior longitudinal ligament

Sacral nerve

Area of periosteum

Anterior sacral foramen

Sacrotuberous ligament

Sacrococcygeal junction

Anterior sacrococcygeal ligament

Figure 4.13. Sacral periosteum and the anterior longitudinal ligament.

Treatment

The pad of the rectal index finger seeks out the periosteal fold or sensitive line. Once there, the finger compresses the line and then follows the Listening. This Induction technique rarely goes beyond a few hundredths of an inch (a few millimeters). Perform this movement several times, increasing the compression little by little. The sensitivity should gradually disappear. This technique provides valuable and long-lasting results.

Precautions

If you encounter a cluster of hemorrhoids, delicately withdraw your finger. Compression of one part of a mass of hemorrhoids can cause a hemorrhoidal thrombus, especially painful in the hours to follow.

Anterior Longitudinal Ligament

This ligament runs from the occiput to the sacrum (fig 4.13). At its sacral attachment it blends with the periosteum. It is often implicated in the trauma known as a "rabbit punch." The resulting fixation prevents the vertebral column from moving smoothly and completely into extension. Freeing up the anterior longitudinal ligament at the sacrum achieves a local pelvic effect and in addition allows the cervical spine to recover its extension. I advise this approach in cases of severe rabbit-punch trauma where direct cervical manipulation is absolutely contraindicated.

This ligament most easily becomes fixated at the transverse ridges that represent the lines of fusion of the vestigial sacral vertebrae. The treatment is the same compression-Induction technique as described for the periosteum.

The Prostate
Initial Approach

The patient lies face-down. Gradually relax the flexion of the intrarectal finger and rotate it internally in such a way that the hand pronates (fig. 4.14). From now on, the pad of the index finger faces ventrally;

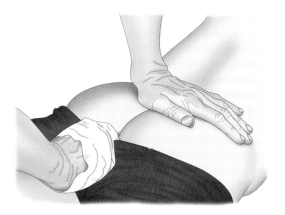

Figure 4.14. Approach to the prostate.

flex the metacarpophalangeal joint to direct the index finger pad caudad. Effect a slight lateral sweep just to the point where the finger meets the prostate. Maintain the index finger deep in the rectum.

Differential Palpation

There is very little risk of error. Occasionally very dry and compacted fecal matter can mislead you. The prostate is a round firm mass about the size of a chestnut. If you go too far in the caudal direction, your finger will feel the pubis, which has the firmness of bone. If you are not sufficiently caudal and ventral, your finger will feel only the rectum.

Advice

In some cases, the prostate is deeply situated and difficult to assess. Ask the patient to place their two fists just above the pubis. In the prone position, their fists will create some pelvic pressure. This pressure naturally brings the prostate closer to your finger.

If palpating the prostate remains difficult, ask the patient to push his buttocks against your finger, as if moving onto all fours. At the same time, push the sacrum caudad with your posterior hand.

Evaluation

Here once again are the parameters to evaluate:

- form and symmetry
- volume
- consistency
- compressibility
- Mobility

- presence of the median sulcus
- sensitivity
- irregularity
- presence of localized hardness

Be careful. If there is ever the slightest doubt, ask your patient to consult a physician. Do not alarm him but simply say that after a certain age it is important to have a routine prostate exam.

Note that 70 percent of prostate cancers occur in the peripheral area, easily accessible by rectal palpation. *Fifty percent of small hardened masses on the prostate, accessible to the finger, turn out to be cancerous.* This underscores the important role an osteopath or manual therapist can play in the detection of prostate cancers. I want to reiterate that whenever you manipulate the sacrococcygeal joint rectally, it is your duty to check the prostate.

Tests
Local Listening Evaluation

Position your index finger pad against the central dorsal part of the prostate. Compress the prostate several times to stimulate its proprioceptive fibers. Release the pressure slightly and allow your finger to move where it is spontaneously and naturally attracted.

Local Listening is not a treatment; it is a way to localize the restriction. The restricted tissues attract your finger. This test allows you to recognize immediately:

- whether there is a fixation or not; if your finger does not move it means there is nothing to manipulate.
- the precise location of a fixation, in which case your finger will move toward the fixation and stop at that level.

▪ the success of you manipulation; the Listening will either have disappeared or be greatly diminished after your treatment. This is proof that you have significantly reduced the tensions.

Mobility Tests

An organ in good health must be mobile. For the prostate it is important to evaluate its anterior-posterior and lateral Mobility. A loss of Mobility particularly affects the prostate's rich venous circulation.

Anterior-Posterior Movement

The rectal index finger pushes the median part of the prostate in a ventral and slightly cranial direction. The prostate does not lie exactly along the longitudinal axis of the body. This is why one tips the testing finger slightly ventrally and caudally rather than mobilizing the prostate in a purely anterior posterior direction. The external hand is placed on the sacrum to push it in a caudal direction, in order to penetrate the finger a little deeper.

Ventral Movement

The first time around, the index finger pad is placed as far cranially as possible. Testing the motion of the prostate in the ventral and cranial directions enables you to evaluate the dorsal cranial structures. Here the extensibility of the rectoprostatic fascia can be appreciated. A fixation of this prostatoperitoneal aponeurosis gives the impression of reduced Mobility accompanied by a slight sensitivity and some crepitation. This test provides information regarding the vesicoprostatic articulation and the seminal vesicles. Any peritoneal fixations can have repercussions for these structures.

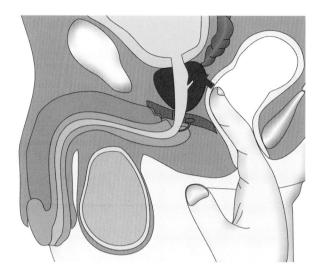

Figure 4.15. Mobility test: ventral movement.

The second time around, repeat the test as above and then glide the index finger caudally. This last action evaluates tensions between the urethra and the prostate.

Compressibility

In this test, the prostate is mobilized against the pubis to appreciate its compressibility. A noncompressible prostate will create undue pressure around the urethra, with all the urinary consequences. Varying the position of the index finger on the prostate allows you to feel the compressibility along the entire length of the organ.

In the case of a fixation between the prostate and the urethra, the patient immediately experiences a strong desire to urinate. This sensation is noteworthy as it should disappear after manipulation. The patient feels the difference as soon as the treatment is over; it is important for him to notice of this change.

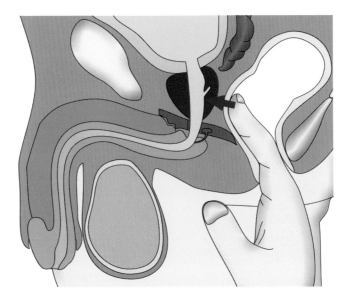

Figure 4.16. The prostate: compression.

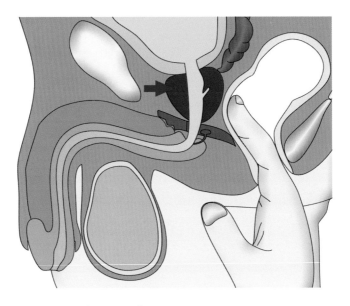

Figure 4.17. The prostate: decompression.

Dorsal Movement

The dorsal Mobility test reveals ventral fixations. Obviously it is impossible for the index finger to move the prostate in a dorsal direction (fig. 4.17); therefore the return movement is evaluated. Push the prostate forward, and then on release, feel whether it immediately regains its initial position. The quality of the return movement is a way to tests the venous plexus of Santorini, the periprostatic sheath, and the pubourethral ligaments. Any resistance to a smooth dorsal return of the prostate indicates a ventral fixation.

Lateral Tests

Transfer your finger to either side of the prostate to mobilize it laterally. These tests are fundamental because the freeing-up of lateral fixations gives the best results in cases of benign prostatic hypertrophy. Lateral Mobility testing demonstrates the extensibility of the sacro-recto-pubic lamina, the levator ani muscles, and the lateral venous plexus. It must be emphasized again that the periprostatic veins are of central concern for manipulation. Because nerve filaments issuing from the hypogastric plexus surround the prostate, lateral fixations can be sensitive when mobilized.

Longitudinal Glide

Place the pad of your index finger centrally on the prostate, initially on its most cranial part and then on its most caudal surface. First, with your finger as cranial as possible, mobilize the prostate in a caudal direction. Inversely, when the finger pad is placed as caudal as possible on the organ, bring the prostate in a cranial direction. This is a global prostate test. Next, with your finger pad on the central part of the prostate, glide the prostate in a caudal and then cranial

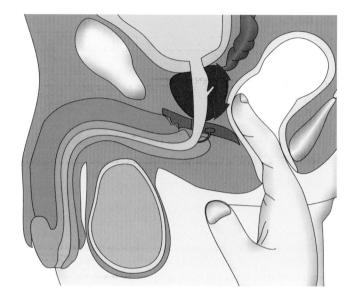

Figure 4.18. Mobility test: longitudinal glide.

direction. This test evaluates extensibility of the urethra and prostate. Fibrosis of the urethra or of the periurethral tissues impedes this up-and-down glide of the prostate.

Manipulation of the Prostate

These manipulations consist of freeing fixations of the prostate and neighboring tissues using direct, indirect, and Induction techniques.

Direct Techniques

The index finger pad contacts fixated areas and mobilizes them in the direction where their Mobility is reduced or absent. For example, if the prostate has a lack of ventral Mobility, the maneuvers would be carried out in a ventral direction. This technique is very effective when the tissues are fibrotic or scarred.

Indirect Techniques

The index finger pad goes in the opposite direction from the area of fixation. It aims to accentuate the Mobility of the free zone. For example, if the prostate has reduced ventral Mobility, you would increase its Mobility in the dorsal direction. For example, take an elbow that lacks flexion; the Indirect Technique mobilizes the joint in extension. Gradually, under the central effect of the mechanoreceptors, the elbow regains its range of motion.

Induction

The finger pad follows the direction of the Listening and exaggerates it. The tissues inform you of the directions to follow.

Be careful: the movement is not just intentional, it is a real mobilization of the tissues in the direction of the Listening. Sometimes Induction takes you in the same direction as the Indirect Technique, but more often the movement is more subtle and follows different axes.

Specific Areas
Seminal Colliculus (Verumontanum)

Recall that the seminal colliculus (fig. 4.19) is a small crest 0.5 inches (1.2 cm) long, 0.04 inches (0.1 cm) wide, and 0.08 inches (0.2 cm) high, where the two ejaculatory ducts open into the prostatic urethra. The seminal colliculus is located in the middle of the inferior prostatic urethral wall.

Prostatic Utricles

The prostatic utricle (fig. 4.19) is situated within the seminal colliculus between the two ejaculatory duct openings. This structure is the vestige of the inferior end of the Müller canals, which give rise to the uterine tubes, uterus, and vagina in women. In men, this structure atrophies completely. The ancients called this uterine homologue the "male vagina," hence the term *utricle*.

Practical Application

It is thought that this region possesses special sensitivity because of its embryological memory. Therefore, manipulation can possibly have an effect on the hormonal system through the prostatic utricle. Recall the discussion above about prostaglandins in the sperm: these hormones relax the uterine neck. This action allows the spermatozoa to pass more easily through the cervical canal. Does manual manipulation play a role in prostaglandin production?

To reach the seminal colliculus in the prostatic urethra, direct your finger pad toward the middle and central part of the prostate.

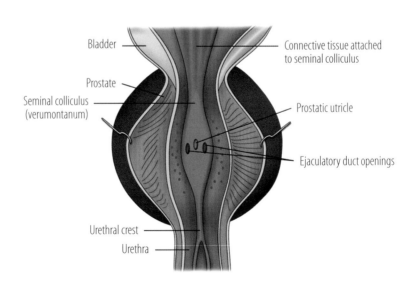

Figure 4.19. Seminal colliculus and prostatic utricle.

Internal Sphincter (Sphincter Vesicae)

At its cranial part, the prostatic urethra is surrounded by smooth muscle fibers that are continuous with the most caudal fibers of the bladder. They surround the urethra and extend into the prostate. This ensemble of fibers forms the smooth-muscle sphincter of the bladder. It is important to manipulate this area because it risks becoming fibrotic and also because of its reflexogenic effect on both the prostate and the bladder.

Protocol

First, apply the Direct Techniques to try to relax the hardened areas as much as possible. Only then embark on the more subtle Induction technique.

Direct Techniques

The Direct Techniques are applied to the urethra and the prostate.

The Urethra
Longitudinal Glide

Glide the pad of your index finger longitudinally in the caudocranial and then craniocaudal direction (fig. 4.18). As a rule, five to six maneuvers is enough. The patient often feels a strong urge to urinate, which should disappear at the end of direct treatment, followed by the Induction technique.

When the posterior median sulcus is present, trace it with your index finger while gradually augmenting your pressure. The goal here is not to mobilize the whole prostate but to stretch the urethra lengthwise.

Transversal Glide

Glide the prostate transversely by placing your finger on either side of the median prostate. Begin at the caudal part and move little by little toward the cranial part of the gland. This is not a global lateral mobilization of the prostate. The goal is the transverse mobilization of the periurethral prostatic tissue.

The Prostate

Compression-Decompression

Here the technique consists of compressing and decompressing the prostate, focusing on any hardened zones. Press the prostate against the pubis and then allow it to regain its normal shape. Repeat this several times (figs. 4.16 and 4.17). This technique seems to have a greater effect on the glandular system of the prostate than on its attachments. However, it does affect the pubovesical ligaments during the decompression phase.

Lateral Lobes

Begin manipulation on the largest and most hardened areas of the hypertrophied lobes. Mobilize the largest area toward the center of the prostate and toward the opposite border. Proceed in this order: first the cephalad part, then the middle area, and finally the caudal part. This maneuver has a double action. It acts on the lateral compressibility of the substance of the prostate, and on the sacro-recto-genito-pubic aponeurosis. It is best always to mobilize both lateral surfaces of the prostate.

Indirect Techniques

The Indirect Techniques are most usefully employed after the Direct Techniques. For example, if the prostate lacks lateral Mobility toward the left, mobilize it fully toward the right. Repeat the Indirect Technique five or six times and then retest the left lateral glide. Very often, the Mobility gain is appreciable. These Indirect Techniques can be carried out on all the components of prostate Mobility.

Induction Technique

Due to the presence of smooth muscle fibers both in the prostate and in the tissues that surround it, this region responds exceptionally well to Induction. Here also the Induction maneuvers are performed on the central part of the prostate, its circumference, and its aponeuroses.

Note that in the urogenital area, as a general rule it is best always to complete treatment with Induction techniques.

Peripheral Part of the Prostate

Apply the same technique on the periphery where the prostate is hardened. First, compress the prostate, release the pressure a little, and then exaggerate the movement of the Listening. The area to be manipulated is shown by the Listening. If your finger is not drawn in a direction, do not force it. The message of the organism is clear.

Around the Prostate
The Prostatoperitoneal Aponeurosis

Direct your index finger as high as possible toward the pouch of Douglas. Release your pressure slightly and treat with Induction. This technique is complementary to the peritoneal technique for the internal inguinal canal. It harmonizes the reciprocal mechanical tensions of the lower part of the peritoneum (fig. 4.20).

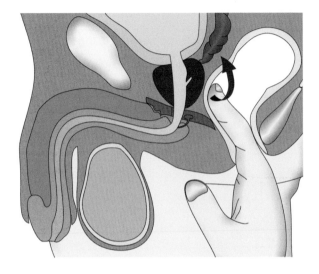

Figure 4.20. Manipulation of the prostatoperitoneal aponeurosis.

The Hypogastric Plexus

The manipulation of this nerve plexus is difficult to distinguish from that of the cranial part of the prostate and the caudal part of the seminal vesicles. The difference lies in directing your index finger laterally. Direct the index finger laterally and then caudally. The sensitivity provoked by approaching the hypogastric plexus confirms the correct location. To differentiate this technique from treatment of the prostatoperitoneal aponeurosis and the seminal vesicles, the finger must stay as far to the lateral as possible. Constantly maintaining the lateral position of the finger, direct it in a somewhat caudocranial direction, searching out a very small sensitive area.

Induction of the Hypogastric Plexus

As with every plexus, Induction achieves the best results. Its effects are measured by decreased pain or sensitivity when touching the prostatic and periprostatic tissues. The improvement can be considerable.

Motility of the Prostate

The index finger compresses the prostate at its most rounded place. Very slowly relax the compression and wait for a very small motion to become apparent. Imagine the shape of the prostate: it is important to have a mental anatomical picture of it (fig. 4.21). The difference between Motility and Listening is subtle but real. It lies in the timing and the movement felt.

Timing

With Listening, the finger is immediately drawn in a direction. With Motility, the movement is slightly delayed.

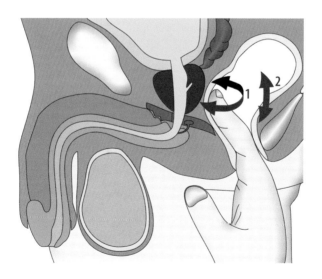

Figure 4.21. Motility of the prostate. 1: Principal motion in rotation. 2: Rarer blotter-type motion.

The Motion

Listening immediately attracts the finger in a single direction and the finger stops at the level of the fixation. Motility is felt under your hand as a slight back and forth rotation around a vertical axis as well as a ventral-dorsal seesaw motion, comparable to cranial flexion-extension.

Effect of Motility

The effect of Motility is felt manually; it is completely subjective. Motility progressively increases in amplitude, intensity, and rhythm (about seven cycles per minute). I believe that Motility has an effect on the vitality of the prostate. When comparing the Motility of a healthy prostate with that of an adenomatous one, the difference is apparent immediately.

The Inguinal Canal

It is important to manipulate the inguinal canal for two reasons: its container and its contents.

The Container

The connections between the inguinal canal and the peritoneum are such that manual manipulation can have a remarkable effect on various peritoneal fixations. These include restrictions due to abdominal scars and trauma as well as hernias of every sort, whether inguinal, umbilical, or hiatal. The inguinal canal is formed by fibers of the internal oblique and secondarily from the external oblique and transversus abdominis. Owing to its essentially muscular formation, the inguinal canal is very receptive to Induction techniques.

The Contents

An effect on the pelvic organs is obtained mainly through the inguinal canal's neural contents. The iliohypogastric, ilioinguinal, and genitofemoral nerves run through the inguinal canal. Methodically evaluate each of these.

Tests

Compare the two inguinal canals in terms of their:

- length
- width
- depth
- resistance

Evaluation of the Inguinal Canal Walls

With your finger placed in the canal, nudge consecutively in these directions:

- lateral
- dorsal
- caudal
- cranial

Gauge the extensibility, elasticity, and sensitivity of the canal walls. Always compare both inguinal canals.

Evaluation of the Inguinal Rings

The openings are surrounded by a fibrous muscular ring whose qualities are to be evaluated:

- hardness
- width
- thickness

To investigate the internal inguinal canal, the palm of your hand brings the homolateral abdominal tissue up against your testing finger in the canal. A fixation gives the impression of being overly tough and is more sensitive.

Evaluation of the Contents

The canal contains the cremaster muscle, testicular vessels, and, of special importance, all the genital branches of the iliohypogastric, inguinal, and iliofemoral nerves. The general sensitivity within the canal provides the most reliable information. It is very difficult to analyze the individual contents of the canal by palpation.

Note: Often a fixation of the inguinal canal at the inguinal ring is accompanied by a fixation of the prostatoperitoneal aponeurosis and the pouch of Douglas on the same side.

Treatment

Induction (fig. 4.22) is the primary inguinal canal technique. Insert the index finger into the canal as if it were entering a thimble. Then exaggerate the movement that you feel in Listening. As a rule you will feel a rotational movement around a large oblique axis from lateral to medial, and from cranial to caudal. These rotations will be clockwise or counterclockwise. The treatment is finished when the finger comes to a standstill.

Apply Induction techniques at the inguinal rings. The internal inguinal ring is a key feature in peritoneal manipulations. While the intrainguinal finger encourages the tissues in Induction, the other hand brings the abdominal tissues to meet it. The external hand carries out Induction as well. It can happen that the two hands find themselves side by side and stretch the tissue together.

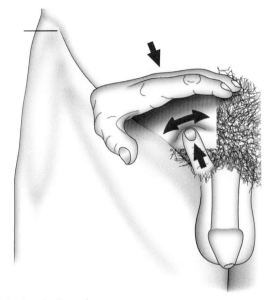

Figure 4.22. Induction of the inguinal canal.

The Seminal Vesicles

Normally it is assumed that the seminal vesicles are inaccessible by rectal palpation. However, I have palpated their caudal part by placing my finger deeply and asking the patient to bring his fists against his pubis to compress the contents of the lesser pelvis. Even though they are deeply situated, it is possible to reach them, especially if they have a problem. When congested and irritated, these structures are larger and more apparent.

Be careful: a seminal vesicle that is painful to the touch or which has a fibrous condition can be indicative of acute or chronic vesiculitis. If the pain is acute, advise your patient to see his doctor. In the case of vesiculitis, the patient feels pain at the end of urination. However, manual therapy is certainly indicated where fibrosity exists. Tests and treatment for the seminal vesicles are outlined below.

Test

The index finger sweeps across the prostate from one lateral border to the other as cranially as possible (fig. 4.23). The prostate feels fairly firm to the touch. When you come across something softer and more depressible, you are on the seminal vesicles. Direct your index finger medially to compress the vesicles; evaluate and compare their compressibility and elasticity. A fixated seminal vesicle is both firmer and more sensitive to the touch.

Treatment

Manipulate in order:

- the prostatoperitoneal aponeurosis
- the pouch of Douglas
- the seminal vesicles

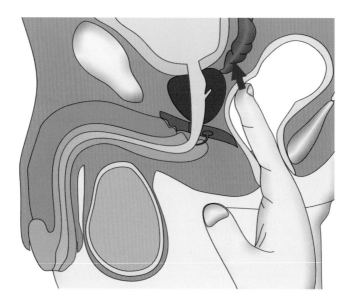

Figure 4.23. Test of the seminal vesicles.

Gently compress the seminal vesicles and perform Induction. As with every paired structure, always compare both sides. Seminal vesicle Motility must exist, but as they are so intimately connected to the bladder, the prostate, and the peritoneum, how can you be sure you are feeling vesicle Motility and not the Motility of one of the other structures?

Cowper's Glands

The Cowper's (bulbourethral) glands are palpable before the anal verge. They are the size of a pea, renitent, and rather compact. Their inflammation manifests outwardly as urethritis. The bulbourethral glands open through minute apertures onto the floor of the urethra. They secrete an alkaline fluid that protects the spermatozoa on their journey from the male urethra to the vagina. They are not the object of specific manipulation.

Ductus Deferens

There are no specific manipulations for these canals either. You have an effect on them in treating the spermatic cord via the inguinal canal. They leave the canal at the deep inguinal ring, where they separate themselves from the other elements of the spermatic cord. They follow the lateral and dorsal surfaces of the bladder, where they become inaccessible. When they reunite at the base of the prostate and contribute to the formation of the ejaculatory ducts, they become manipulable once again.

Remember the target zone of the seminal colliculus. It is the place where the ejaculatory canals expel semen into the urethra at approximately the middle inferior part of the prostate.

Effects of Manipulation

Results vary from patient to patient as the effects of manipulation depend on the original problem. The therapist will feel a difference in the tissues he or she palpates. To the extent that results are noticed by the patient, they most commonly report an improvement in urinary problems.

Palpation

- The prostate is more mobile, more compressible, and elastic.
- The urethra is less fibrous and more extensible.
- The seminal vesicles are suppler and less sensitive.
- Compressing the urethra during palpation no longer causes the urge to urinate.
- The prostate is rarely diminished in size.

Symptoms

The patient notices improvement in urinary function:

- less urgency
- less getting up to urinate during the night
- a more powerful and consistent stream
- an increase in bladder autonomy
- easier ejaculation—typically patients speak less willingly about this problem
- fewer infectious episodes of chronic prostatitis

Chapter 5

A Global Approach

The Principle of Global Lesion

Respecting this principle means not being content with local manipulation alone. All pelvic structures have links with the rest of the body, including the abdomen, thorax, cranium, or periphery. The special relationship between the prostate and the left kidney is described above, for example. Certain tissue associations are commonly found, and they will be touched on here.

The Lower Extremities

Nearly all the muscles and aponeuroses of the thigh have a connection with the container and contents of the lesser pelvis. However, the biceps muscle of the femur merits special mention.

Fixation of the Fibula

The biceps femoris muscle shares fibers with the ligaments that join the sacrum to the ischium. The sacrotuberous and sacrospinous ligaments are veritable witnesses to all homolateral visceral problems. Fibers of these ligaments continue into the tendon of the long head of the biceps femoris. Thus a visceral fixation will create abnormal tension on the biceps femoris muscle, which will in turn pull on its fibular insertion. In systematically testing the head of the fibula in the majority of patients, it is astonishing how frequently a unilateral

fibular fixation is discovered. When questioned, these patients sel-
dom report having sustained a trauma to the area. *In effect, a fixation
of the head of the fibula, without antecedent trauma, is often of visceral origin.* One quality that these fixations share is their ready tendency to
change after homolateral visceral fixations are resolved.

Fixations of the First and Fifth Metatarsals

The peroneus longus muscle attaches to the head of the fibula. This
muscle is subject to any abnormal tension of the biceps femoris muscle, and this continuity will affect its distal attachment at the first
metatarsal. Likewise, the peroneus brevis also suffers the consequences of these myofascial tensions, which come to bear on its distal attachment at the fifth metatarsal.

The Proprioceptive System of the Foot

The arch of the foot is an eminently reflexogenic zone for the viscera
and the proprioceptive system. On the bottom of each foot are seven
thousand nerve receptors linking the plantar arch to the brain. In a
millionth of a second these nerves must inform the cerebellum about
the foot's relationship to the ground. A visceral fixation can perturb
these mechanoreceptors and cause a sprain, for example. The foot
has three major weight-bearing points of contact: the calcaneous, the
first metatarsal, and the fifth metatarsal bones. If, through the myofascial chains, the first and fifth metatarsals become fixated, it is easy
to understand why proprioception becomes distorted.

A foot fixation is sometimes simply due to a myofascial imbalance coming from an intrapelvic organ. When the myofascial chain
has abnormal tension, the proprioceptive system not only fails to

send the correct information to the brain, it also delays the immediate retroactive response from the nervous system. As a result, when the foot steps on the ground, the appropriate muscular contractions are not made in time, and a sprain occurs.

Manipulating an organ can have an effect on the equilibrium dynamics of the foot and vice versa.

The Liver

The relationship of the liver to the prostate's considerable venous system means this organ must be treated.

Mechanically:

- Treat the liver's attachments: the left triangular ligament, the coronary ligament, and the falciform ligament.
- Manipulate the organ itself by compression-decompression and Induction.

Counsel the patient to promote a healthy liver:

- Encourage him in physical activity.
- Advise the patient to avoid alcohol, tobacco, chocolate, spices, fats, animal protein, and salt.
- Ask him to eat more vegetables (broccoli, tomatoes), fruits (lemon, papaya), and sunflower, canola, and flax-seed oils.
- Suggest he take zinc, selenium, and flax seeds as supplements.
- Recommend he drink water with a few drops of lemon added. This should be sipped frequently during the day, but just a little at a time. Also, decongestant herbal teas (nettle tea, for example) are beneficial.

Often men who have benign prostatic hypertrophy drink as little as possible to avoid the inherent urinary problems. As a result, they eliminate fewer toxins and lose their vitality. It is good to be clear with them about the drawbacks of such behavior and suggest they change their habits little by little. They follow this kind of advice more willingly when they notice a rapid improvement in their condition.

Chapter 6
The Emotional Plane

Some organs are clearly linked to one's way of life and to particular stresses. The stomach responds to relational stress, the "social me" that manages our relations with others and with society around us. On the emotional plane, the prostate is subtle to interpret. In any event, when it comes to psychoemotional problems, one enters the subjective realm and speaks more of tendencies than of certitudes.

It has been observed that vulnerability to BPH is greatest around fifty to sixty years of age, presumably due to hormonal changes. This modification often coincides with a socioprofessional change.

Changes in Social Life

For some men, this is the age when they must leave their jobs. They may fear a loss of influence and descent into anonymity. In earlier times, the prostate was sometimes referred to as the "beacon." Remember that the word *prostate* comes from the Greek meaning "placed in front" but also "to be exposed." It is the beacon that permits us to see and also to be exposed before others. In quitting work, a man can think that he will lose his role as a beacon and with it the recognition of others.

Women have traditionally had at least two strong poles of attraction: their work and their homes. Men—generalizing here, of course—traditionally have often had only their work. If a man takes separation from the world of work badly, he can become depressed. The prostate will be one of the organs targeted by this depression.

Returning Home

For some men, the return to home life is not simple. To go from having a certain social status at work to being an everyday homebody is sometimes difficult to accept. The richer and more captivating his professional life, the more problematic his retirement can prove to be.

Traditionally, as a rule, women have managed the household. At first a man may oppose her in trying to find his new place. Such confrontation becomes a source of conflict. Happily, with time each partner gradually establishes their territory and role. During this period, however, divorce rates increase. If the conflict goes on for too long, the tension compounds the depression that may have arisen from leaving work, and prostate problems are worsened. This description is, of course, only a generalization, but in questioning the people around you, you might be surprised at how common such stories are.

Solitude

Allow the patient to describe his life, whatever it was and whatever it is yet to become. Often, he expresses true anguish by asking you, "What shall I make of my life now?" This simple crisis of conscience indicates that he has already taken an important step. Sometimes a patient will ask if he should seek counseling, and this too signifies that a part of the work has already been done.

Men are often profoundly reticent to talk willingly talk about urinary symptoms, or if they do, it is with derision. Knowing how to listen tactfully is perhaps more important than you might think. This is a service osteopaths and manual therapists must also provide.

Conclusion

Osteopathy and manual therapy are slowly becoming an incontrovertible element of health care. I can say with pride that almost all babies in my area, France, have seen an osteopath or manual therapist, mostly on prophylactic grounds.

The prostate and related techniques described here are effective. As osteopaths and manual therapists we must use them, especially preventively, if we are to carry out our social role fully. Prostate problems are arising with increasing frequency. Part of our power as osteopaths and manual therapists is to help delay or avoid surgery. It is up to us to take on this role. While we have already gone some distance, the road ahead is still long.

Glossary

Adenoma of the prostate: benign hypertrophy or hyperplasia of the prostate gland.

Alpha-blockers: drugs that block the response of alpha-adrenergic receptors that circulate adrenaline secreted by the central nervous system. These medications reduce the tone of smooth muscle fibers and are used, for example, to relax the bladder neck.

Androgens: steroid hormones that increase the development of male genitalia, spermatogenesis, and secondary male sexual characteristics. Ninety percent of this anabolic protein stimulant is produced in the testicles and 10 percent comes from the adrenal glands.

Anuria: a decline in urinary output resulting in absence of urine in the bladder.

Apyrexia: absence or remission of fever.

BPH: benign prostatic hypertrophy. See *prostatic adenoma.*

Colles's ligament (reflected inguinal ligament): made up of fibers of the external oblique aponeurosis coming from the opposite side. Forms the caudal part of the external pillar of the external inguinal ring.

Conjoint tendon: the merging of the pubic attachments of the internal oblique and transverse abdominal aponeuroses into a common tendon.

Cowper's glands: two small bulbourethral glands, located either side of the prostate and draining to the urethra. They secrete an alkaline fluid.

Cremaster muscle: draws the testis up toward the superficial inguinal ring. The cremaster arises from the inguinal ligament and accompanies the spermatic cord through the inguinal canal.

Crural arch: a tough fibrous sheath running from the anterior superior iliac spine to the pubic spine.

Direct Technique: manipulation in the direction against the mechanical resistance of a tissue.

Diuresis: increased secretion of urine by the kidney.

Ductus deferens: this canal arises from the tail of the epididymis of the testis, ascends from the scrotum, and joins the seminal vesicle to form the ejaculatory canal. It passes through the inguinal canal as a component of the spermatic cord.

Dysuria: painful or difficult urination.

Epididymis: small oblong grayish bodies lying on the superior part of the testicle. These paired ducts carry sperm from the seminiferous tubules of the testis to the ductus deferens.

Escherichia coli (E. coli): a species of the coliform bacteria of the Enterobacteriaceae family. *E. coli* is the most frequent cause of urinary tract infection.

Excretion: expulsion of substances by organs or tissues.

Gimbernat's (lacunar) ligament: an extension from the deep aspect of the inguinal ligament to the pectineal line, this ligament forms the floor of the inguinal canal. It is a fibrous sheath filling in the acute angle formed by the internal crural arcade and the pecten pubis.

Hesselbach's triangle (also known as the inguinal triangle): region of the abdominal wall defined by the following structures: rectus abdominis muscle (medially), inferior epigastric vessels (superiorly and laterally), inguinal ligament (inferiorly).

Hydrocele: an accumulation of serous fluid in the tunica vaginalis (the visceral layer surrounding the testicle) or in the fascia along the spermatic cord.

Hydronephrosis: dissension of the pelvis and calyces of the kidney by urine that cannot flow past an obstruction in the ureter. Swelling and sensitivity in the kidney result.

Iliopectineal band: part of the iliac fascia that runs from the crural arch to the pectineal line.

Indirect Technique: manipulation in the opposite direction of the mechanical tissue fixation; direction of ease.

LH: luteinizing hormone.

LH-RH: luteinizing hormone–releasing hormone.

Ligament of Henle: reinforcement of the transversalis fascia between the external border of the rectus abdominis and the internal inguinal ring.

Ligament of Hesselbach: reinforcements of the transversalis fascia that join the crural arch.

Manual Induction technique: Induction is the exaggeration of tissue Listening in order to manipulate a tissue fixation.

Manual tissue Listening: the passive attraction of the hand toward a tissue fixation.

Mycoplasma: bacteria causing prostatitis.

Neck of the prostate: distal and caudal part of the prostate.

Oligospermia: insufficient spermatozoa in the semen.

Oligosthenospermia: reduction in number and Mobility of spermatozoa.

Pectineal (Cooper's) ligament: a thick, dense, and fibrous cord running from the spine of the pubis to the iliopectineal line.

Pollakiuria: unduly frequent passage of small quantities of urine.

Polyuria: excretion of abnormally large quantities of urine in a day.

Prostate specific antigen (PSA): enzyme secreted by the prostate gland responsible, among other things, for the fluidity of sperm. A protein produced in minute quantities by the prostate cells, but at elevated levels by cancerous cells.

Pyuria: presence of pus in the urine.

Retrograde ejaculation: an ejaculation of semen in a reverse direction, back toward the bladder.

Scrotum: skin containing the testicles.

Seminal colliculus (verumontanum): small longitudinal median elevation on the posterior wall of the prostatic urethra. The prostatic
utricle and the ejaculatory ducts open onto the seminal colliculus.

Smooth sphincter: surrounds the origin of the prostatic urethra. It is
continuous with the trigone of the bladder.

Sperm (semen): secretion of the various male reproductive organs:
testicles, epididymis, seminal vesicles, prostate, and bulbourethral
glands.

Striated sphincter: located at the caudal part of the prostatic urethra.

Stroma: the vascularized connective tissue matrix of an organ (as dis-
tinguished from its parenchyma). It is the supporting tissue of an
organ, gland, or tumor. The stroma of the prostate comprises muscular fibers.

Tissue fixation: loss of tissue Mobility, extensibility, or elasticity.

Transurethral prostate resection: prostatectomy without removal of the
prostatic capsule.

Utricle: small pouch situated on the median line of the prostatic urethra. It opens onto the seminal colliculus.

Varicocele: dilatation of the pampiniform venous complex of the
spermatic veins, most commonly on the left. This manifests at the
caudal part of the scrotum, often accompanied by hernia, hemorrhoids, and varicosities of the lower extremities.

Vesical blockage: extremely painful acute urine retention.

Bibliography

Bates, B. *Guide de l'examen clinique.* Paris: Medsi-Edisem, 1980.

Croibier, A. Personal notes. Meylan, France, 2002.

Debré, B., with P. Evevrad, A. Maeur, and J. P. Abecassis. *Tout savoir sur la prostate.* Paris: Favre, 2001.

Dousset, H. *L'Examen du malade en clientèle.* Paris: Maloine, 1964.

Flam, T., with D. Amsellem-Ouazana, A. Ameur, and E. Husson. *Mémento d'urologie.* Paris: Maloine, 2002.

Fritsch, H., and W. Kuhnel. *Atlas de poche d'anatomie.* Paris: Flammarion-Médecine-Sciences, 2007.

Kahle, W., H. Leonhardt, and W. Platzer. *Anatomie 1: Appareil locomoteur.* Paris: Flammarion-Médecine-Sciences, 1982.

Kahle, W., H. Leonhardt, and W. Platzer. *Anatomie 2: Viscères.* Paris: Flammarion-Médecine-Sciences, 1978.

Kahle, W., H. Leonhardt, and W. Platzer. *Anatomie 3: Système nerveux.* Paris: Flammarion-Médecine-Sciences, 1981.

Lazorthes, G. *Le Système nerveux périphérique.* Paris: Masson, 1971.

Ligner, B. Personal notes. Annecy, France, 1987.

Prat, D. Personal notes. La Grive, France, 1999.

Rommeveaux, L. Personal notes. Proveysieux, France, 2000.

Silbernagl, S., and A. Despopoulos. *Atlas de poche de physiologie, 4e ed.* Paris: Flammarion-Médecine-Sciences, 1992.

Testut, L., and O. Jacob. *Traité d'anatomie topographique.* Paris: Doin, 1922.

Testut, L., and A. Latarjet. *Appareil uro-génitalpéritoine.* Paris: Doin, 1931.

Index

Transversalis fascia, 30, 38

Transverse rectal fold, 5

Transversus abdominis muscle,
28, 38

Tunica vaginalis, 35, 37

About the Author

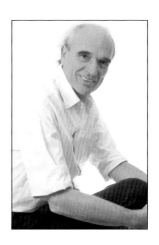

Named by *Time* magazine as one of the top healing innovators to watch in the new millennium, Jean-Pierre Barral, DO, MRO(F), RPT, is an osteopath and registered physical therapist who serves as director and faculty member of the Department of Osteopathic Manipulation at the University of Paris School of Medicine in France. He is a member of the Registre des Ostéopathes de France. He also holds a diploma of the Faculty of Medicine of Paris North, one of only four osteopaths in the world to hold such a diploma. Trained at the European School of Osteopathy in Maidstone, England, he has authored many manual therapy textbooks, including *Visceral Manipulation* (Eastland Press 1988, 2005) and *Manual Therapy for the Peripheral Nerves* (Elsevier 2004, 2007). He has also written a trade book for the general public titled *Understanding the Messages of Your Body: How to Interpret Physical and Emotional Signals to Achieve Optimal Health* (North Atlantic Books, 2007). He developed the modality of Visceral Manipulation which is a manual therapy that focuses on the internal organs, their environment, and their potential influence on many structural and physiological dysfunctions. His approach has been taught to over ten thousand practitioners worldwide through the Barral Institute (www.barralinstitute.com) in West Palm Beach, Florida.